THRUSH

Other titles in this series:
Bladder Problems
Osteoporosis
Smear Tests

THRUSH

The Yeast Infection You Can Beat

Jane Butterworth

Thorsons
An Imprint of HarperCollinsPublishers

Thorsons
An Imprint of HarperCollins*Publishers*
77–85 Fulham Palace Road,
Hammersmith, London W6 8JB

Published by Thorsons 1991
3   5   7   9   10   8   6   4   2

A CIP catalogue record for this book
is available from the British Library

ISBN 0 7225 2503 6

Typeset by Harper Phototypesetters Limited,
Northampton, England
Printed in Great Britain by
HarperCollinsManufacturing, Glasgow

CONTENTS

Introduction   7

1: What On Earth Is It?   9
2: Why Does It Happen?   17
3: What Else Could It Be?   31
4: What Doctors Can Do   45
5: Naturally Good Health   55
6: How To Handle Stress   63
7: Strengthening Your Body's Defences   73
8: You Are What You Eat: Thrush and Diet   83
9: Acupuncture and Bodily Harmony   91
10: The Healing Power of Herbs   99
11: Keeping Thrush At Bay – For Good   109

Further Reading   121
Useful Addresses   123
References   125
Index   127

INTRODUCTION

W HAT IS IT ABOUT THRUSH that makes it so distressing? It is a common affliction that has no serious medical complications, and yet it causes immense anguish to so many women.

All vaginal infections are wretched. They can make us feel ashamed and unclean. They can undermine our sexuality and sap our confidence. After all, they affect an intimate part of our body which is usually reserved only for lovers.

Thrush is particularly insidious because, just as you think you've got rid of it, it can return with a vengeance. An unlucky few of us will suffer attacks as often as once a month, which can be emotionally debilitating. Relationships have broken down under the strain.

It was significant that every woman I spoke to, without exception, had experienced thrush in varying degrees of severity. Many of them had their own special ways of coping with the problem, and provided me with valuable information. A special thanks to all the friends who helped me by recalling their experiences, extracts from which I've included throughout the text.

Thrush seems even more alarming when you know nothing about it. Many women wrongly believe it is a sexually transmitted disease, and because of this are too ashamed or afraid to seek treatment. Yet thrush can not only be treated, but controlled.

7

This book looks at the various ways you can treat thrush and prevent it from recurring, by using a range of orthodox or complementary treatments. It includes self-help remedies to treat symptoms and prevent further attacks, and pays special attention to diet, way of life and stress management.

If the book achieves its aim, it will dispel a lot of the myths which surround this disagreeable complaint, and help you to enjoy a thrush-free existence.

Chapter 1

WHAT ON EARTH IS IT?

Can there be worse sickness than to know
That we are never well, nor can be so?

JOHN DONNE

M OST WOMEN'S FIRST REACTION on learning they have thrush is: what on earth is it?

Thrush, or monilia as it used to be called, is a yeast-like fungal infection caused by an organism called *Candida albicans*, which is naturally present in most of us. Normally, the organism lives quite happily in our intestines and vagina along with a lot of other bacteria. When we're healthy and our immune system is functioning properly, the yeast is kept under control by the friendly bacteria with which it shares its home, and by the natural acidity of the vagina. But if anything compromises our immune system or disturbs the harmony of our intestinal or vaginal bacteria, the yeast can start to grow out of control. Soon it will manifest itself as a fungal infection, not unlike athlete's foot.

The vagina is protected by lactic bacteria, most notably *Lactobacillus acidophilus*. Lactic bacteria are our 'friendly' vaginal flora: they are micro-organisms which are normally present in the skin, the intestines, and the vagina, and their role is to transform sugars into lactic acid. The vaginal walls secrete glycogen, a sugar compound, and when our bodies are in good health, the lactic bacteria act on the glycogen. The result is a slightly acidic environment which works well at keeping harmful micro-organisms and yeasts under control.

The balance is delicate, and if anything disturbs that balance by destroying the lactic bacteria from the digestive system or the vagina, or by making the vaginal secretions more alkaline/less acidic (the desirable level is pH4.5, which is acidic), the yeast can start to grow out of control.

Vaginal thrush is a complaint which women only normally develop in the years between the menarche (the onset of periods) and the menopause, which is often a consoling thought for recurrent sufferers. This is because after the menopause, there is not enough vaginal sugar to ensure the growth of the yeast, unless the woman is receiving hormone replacement therapy.

The first time thrush is diagnosed can be confusing and even alarming. Many women are repelled at the thought of a fungus growing in their vagina. Questions flood through their mind: is it a sexually transmitted disease? Can my partner catch it? What will happen if I don't get treated? Will it return again? Does it mean I am unclean? What's the best way of treating it? And how can I get rid of it for good?

Discovering that it is the commonest female problem second only to anaerobic bacterial vaginosis (see page 39) in the US and that 75 per cent of us[1] will suffer from it at least once in our adult lives is reassuring. But although thrush rarely results in hospitalization or indeed has any serious repercussions at all, that doesn't make us feel any better when we develop it.

Any vaginal infection can be traumatic and cause a considerable amount of distress. As a society, we have taboos about female genitals: unlike men, we go to the lavatory in private, we shrink from discussing problems connected with them, and we tend to be almost fanatically fastidious about keeping them clean. So when we do develop a genital disorder, we have a tendency to think of ourselves as unclean.

A quarter of us will go through life and never develop thrush. Out of the remainder, most will have occasional attacks which will respond quickly to treatment, but a relatively small but unfortunate number of women will have recurrent chronic attacks of thrush – some as often as once a month.

The widespread use of antibiotics is probably the commonest cause of thrush. At best, antibiotics are lifesavers, but they are frequently abused, and often it's ourselves, the patients, who are to blame. Every time we have a sore throat or a slight infection, instead of letting our bodies heal it naturally, which is what will happen eventually, we become impatient. We want an instant cure – and so we go to our doctor and demand antibiotics.

The trouble is, antibiotics not only efficiently polish off the harmful bacteria, they kill the good bacteria, too: that same bacteria we've just seen is so essential to protect the vagina against infections and yeast overgrowth. There are other factors, too, which can upset the harmony of your vaginal flora and provoke thrush as we shall see in the following chapters: stress, disease, poor nutrition, perfumed soaps, bubble baths and vaginal deodorants, a weak immune system – even the clothes you wear. The pH level in the vagina can be raised from its slightly acidic normal level of 4.5 by a number of factors including menstruation and pregnancy, and the resulting alkaline environment provides an excellent breeding ground for the yeast to grow.

In order for our friendly bacteria to flourish and provide an antidote to the yeast organism, our immune system must be strong and our diet needs to include lactose (milk sugar), complex carbohydrates, vitamin C and fibre to encourage the bacteria to grow. If not, and in particular if lactose is lacking, they will die and yeasts can start to grow.

Although thrush can also appear in the mouth, particularly in children, and in other parts of the body, the vagina is the ideal fungal host – it's warm, damp, and dark. And once the yeast starts to grow, it grows rapidly, particularly if you're nourishing it by eating a diet high in sugar and yeast-based foods. The demand for fast food has led to many of us consuming a diet high in starch and sugar which provides the ideal breeding ground for the thrush spores. It's easy to see why thrush has become so prevalent.

Once established, the *candida* organism can be obstinately

difficult to shift. Orthodox medicine usually consists of anti-fungals which clear up the symptoms, but it can recur: one study found that about a quarter of the women whose thrush cleared up after such treatment were found to have positive vaginal cultures again within 30 days,[2] which suggests that the only way to rid ourselves of thrush effectively is to treat the cause, not the symptoms. It is at this that we will be looking in the following chapters.

Although Hippocrates, who is recognized in the West as being the father of medicine, referred to thrush as early as 2,000 years ago, vaginal thrush was probably very rare in the days when our ancestors wore no knickers and long, loose skirts. Thrush thrives in the sort of nice warm conditions our modern clothes create for them: close-fitting knickers, tights, and jeans, especially if they are made from man-made fibres, trap heat and provide an ideal environment for thrush.

Often thrush and cystitis join together to form a ghastly vicious circle, with one regularly following the other, and that really can be distressing. Swimming regularly in public swimming baths which are cleaned with chlorine can also trigger off thrush. It is paradoxical that many women think of thrush as an unclean affliction, because obsessive cleanliness can make it worse. The first thing many women do at the first sign of thrush is to jump in a bath, yet hot baths only exacerbate the problem because they provide the yeast with a warm wet environment in which to grow.

Many women are ashamed to admit they have thrush because they perceive it as a sexually transmitted disease. They fear that people might think they have contracted it because they are promiscuous. But you can't 'catch' thrush. It usually occurs spontaneously, whether you have a sexual partner or not. You can get thrush if you have been strictly monogamous, celibate, or have multiple partners. You can get it if your partner wears a condom. Thrush can also be passed on by hand, and since it thrives in the mouth as well, can affect children, too. Occasionally it can be passed on through oral sex.

Men and Thrush

However, men can be affected by your thrush, and it can lead to them developing their own form of thrush – balanitis, an acute inflammation under the foreskin which is occasionally accompanied by a discharge. It is rare for a man to develop this unless their female partner has vaginal thrush, or unless the man is diabetic. Up to 25 per cent of the male partners of women with thrush can carry the yeast spores without showing symptoms at all.[3] Some men can also develop a hypersensitive reaction which usually consists of itching and inflammation, but the symptoms usually only last an hour or so after intercourse. Uncircumcised men are more prone to balanitis.

So even though it's not really a sexually transmitted disease, it's a good idea to refrain from sex during an attack. Apart from the possibility that you may transmit yeast spores to your partner, sex can aggravate an infection. It makes sense for the male partners of women with thrush to seek treatment as well, because if they don't there's a chance they can set off another thrush attack in their partner.

What Are the Symptoms?

The chances are that by now you're familiar with at least one of the symptoms of thrush. The most usual symptom is a thick white curdy discharge that is often likened to cottage cheese, although it can be watery. This is usually accompanied by a maddening itching around the vulval area (the outer genitals) or vagina, and there is sometimes a rather disagreeable yeast-like smell. The vagina can be red and inflamed, and the vulval area can look swollen and inflamed. Passing urine can hurt like mad. Sex can also become painful. If you've got all those symptoms, the thrush has really got established.

If you've never had thrush before, you must go and see a doctor to get it properly diagnosed. Don't attempt self-diagnosis: there are many vaginal infections, as we shall see in chapter 3, with which thrush shares similar symptoms, and some of them can have serious repercussions if left untreated. Often thrush is accompanied by other diseases whose symptoms can be masked by the thrush.

A doctor can only diagnose thrush accurately if he or she takes swabs for analysis: a diagnosis of thrush just by physical examination is not always accurate. After the initial attack, most women recognize the early signs of thrush. In the following chapters we will be looking at some precautions you can take if you think a thrush attack is imminent, to try and stop the yeast from taking hold.

Because thrush is a relatively minor complaint, some women tend to suffer it in silence, because they don't want to bother their doctor about it. Sometimes they can be too embarrassed to seek help because they don't like discussing complaints of an intimate nature with a male doctor. What makes it harder, too, is that because, medically speaking, thrush is a minor complaint, some doctors don't give it the attention it deserves. In chapter 4 we will look at the various options available to you if you believe you are not getting the attention from your doctor you deserve.

It is essential that thrush is properly diagnosed and treated because it can occasionally lead to other, more serious complaints. Often it can appear with other conditions, like cystitis and trichomonas. If it persists, it can be an indicator of a severely impaired immune system. But most of all it should be treated because if left unchecked, it can be depressing, distressing and spoil your sexual enjoyment. So don't be shy about seeking help.

Vaginal infections develop easily and can be difficult to get rid of. This is because women's bodies aren't going to win any design prizes: frankly, we're rather poorly constructed in the pelvic area. We are constantly at risk of infecting ourself with harmful rectal bacteria every time we go to the lavatory, because the vagina is situated right in the middle of the urethra, which carries urine from the bladder to outside the body, and the rectum, which carries waste from the body's intestines.

Unless you are scrupulous about hygiene, the rectal bacteria can be a constant source of infection to the vagina or urethra, as many cystitis sufferers know to their cost. Because these orifices are so close to each other, it doesn't take much imagination to realize how easily germs can be passed from one to the other.

Candida allowed to flourish unchecked will keep recurring and eventually could start presenting other seemingly unrelated symptoms. Tiredness, bloatedness, depression, food cravings, digestive problems and recurrent sore throats are just a few symptoms which could be a result of a severe infestation with candida. Make sure it doesn't happen to you. By making a few changes to your life you can prevent the yeast from flourishing and stop thrush from recurring.

Knowledge is power. It gives us the ability and confidence to make our own decisions, rather than allow doctors to make them for us. Ignorance is not only bewildering, it makes us vulnerable and puts us at the mercy of a medical profession which is not always motivated by altruism. Knowledge gives us choice. The more we know about thrush, the more options for treatment we have at our disposal. We can choose what form of treatment suits us best as individuals, rather than be told what somebody else thinks is best.

This book should enable you to make your own choices about how to control your thrush. In the next chapter we will be looking at what factors aggravate thrush; what sort of people are predisposed to getting it; and why it happens.

Chapter 2

WHY DOES IT HAPPEN?

*C*ANDIDA SPECIES can be recovered in virtually any part of a healthy human body. It's in the vagina even when there is no sign of thrush: it is only when something happens to precipitate it that the organism can grow out of control and set up a fungal infection.

Normally, *candida* is kept in check by the body's immune system. When the immune system is working well, as soon as the yeast organism starts trying to grow beyond its normal sites the body's defences attack and destroy it. But if the immune system is weak, and if there are a number of other predisposing factors – an alkaline environment, a diet high in carbohydrates – then the fungus can grow out of control.

To see how vaginal thrush can occur, we must start by having a look at what's going on in the vagina.

The vagina is constantly producing mucus. Some women become alarmed when they notice discharge stains on their underwear, but vaginal secretions are perfectly normal. Our vaginas need secretions to keep them clean and healthy in much the same as our mouths need saliva.

The vagina is rather like a collapsed tube. Its walls are normally like folds of skin which can expand to accommodate a penis or a baby, and it is always moist. However, depending on your age and at what stage you are in your cycle, it can vary from being fairly moist to very wet.

The vaginal secretions not only keep the vagina lubricated but they also keep it clean and free from germs. The cervix also produces its own mucus according to the different stages of the menstrual cycle, and together with the vaginal secretions this forms a slightly acidic environment which can destroy harmful bacteria.

A healthy vagina is constantly producing milky secretions that are slightly acidic, and often have a distinctive sweetish smell. The quantity and consistency varies enormously from person to person, and also depends on what stage of the menstrual cycle you are at, for the female sex hormones oestrogen and progesterone are responsible for producing the secretions. Each month we secrete oestrogen and progesterone in varying amounts throughout our cycle, and these secretions are essential to our health and well-being.

The normal vaginal mucus is different from the copious amounts of lubricating fluid which are secreted by the lower part of the vagina when we are sexually aroused. If the vagina is dry during sex it is not only uncomfortable and painful, but it is also liable to become irritated, or tear and become open to infection.

What's Normal?

As ovulation approaches, the consistency and quantity of the discharge changes. You should become more aware of it as it becomes more copious, and it is clearer and stretchier. When ovulation occurs, the discharge sometimes becomes clear and jelly-like, because of the changes in the cervical mucus, which make it easier for the sperm to enter the womb and fertilize the egg. After ovulation, the discharge usually becomes scantier until the pre-menstrual period when, due to the fall in the hormone progesterone which heralds the start of menstruation, there could be another few days of fairly profuse, watery discharge. Secretions increase if your oestrogen level is high or if you are under emotional stress.

The vaginal secretions maintain the acidity of the vagina and this helps prevent infection. A slightly acid vagina discourages the growth of unwanted organisms like *candida*. This is why pre-menstrual thrush is common, for menstrual blood raises the pH level of the vagina, creating the sort of alkaline environment which provides a good breeding ground for thrush.

Oestrogen is responsible for glycogen (sugar) to be deposited in the vaginal cells. Sometimes the level of oestrogen can increase – during pregnancy, or as a result of taking some sorts of contraceptive pill, or because of a hormone imbalance – and this can result in an increased amount of vaginal sugar. As we saw in the previous chapter, our vaginal bacteria level is finely balanced, and if anything disturbs that balance then the yeast can start to grow out of control. A surfeit of sugar can cause this to happen.

Only you really know what's normal for you. Some women have quite a heavy normal discharge; others have only a very slight white stain. What's normal is that the same pattern is repeated, month after month. A normal discharge may stain underwear but is not normally so profuse that sanitary protection needs to be worn. It shouldn't smell unpleasant – indeed, many men find the smell attractive – and it is painless except on occasions when some women experience slight twinges at the time of their ovulation.

It's absolutely normal to see a small whitish stain on your underwear each day. That's the colour the mucus becomes when it comes into contact with oxygen. If you get to know your body, you can learn exactly at which stage of your menstrual cycle you are at simply by examining the discharge: some women use this as a form of natural contraception.

A discharge isn't normal when it's different from usual. When it's so profuse you have to wear protection, or is an unpleasant colour, or it smells offensive, or is accompanied by itching, pain or any sort of discomfort, it could indicate an infection is present.

Antibiotics

Probably the most common reason for the increase in thrush is the widespread use of broad spectrum antibiotics. Antibiotics – penicillin, streptomycin and tetracycline are just some well known brands – are drugs used to treat infections caused by bacteria and similar organisms. They are not effective against viruses, which cause colds, flu, most respiratory infections and sore throats.

They were derived from living organisms which prevent the growth of other organisms; for example, the drug penicillin is made from the mould *Penicillium*, and it kills off a variety of bacteria – indeed, many of us owe our lives to this remarkable drug.

But antibiotics should not be used indiscriminately. Long-term treatment with the same antibiotic increases the chance of the growth of drug-resistant organisms, which is an important reason for using these drugs sparingly. They also cost health services a great deal of money every year. But what is of most interest to thrush sufferers is that they can kill off the harmless 'friendly' bacteria that normally live in the intestine and the vagina, as well as the harmful bacteria they are intended to kill.

We've already talked about how essential *Lactobacillus acidophilus*, our 'friendly' vaginal bacteria, is to our good health. It's responsible for transforming vaginal sugars into lactic acid, and keeping the vaginal secretions acidic enough to prevent the harmful yeasts and bacteria from multiplying.

If antibiotics kill off our friendly bacteria, the conditions in our vagina become unbalanced. Without anything to control it, the yeast that lives in us begins to thrive and grow, and eventually manifests itself as a fungal infection. Not only that, antibiotics can weaken our immune system which has probably already been weakened by the infection which has necessitated the taking of antibiotics in the first place.

It's important only to take antibiotics when you have a severe infection – not for trivial afflictions like a sore throat. Most doctors nowadays do only prescribe antibiotics when strictly necessary, and there are, of course, times when antibiotics are essential. If you have suffered from thrush in the past you should tell your doctor and ask if there is any other treatment available.

Most doctors will suggest taking a course of anti-fungals such as nystatin simultaneously with antibiotics. But as we shall see in chapter 3, the trouble with anti-fungals is that they treat the symptoms and not the cause – and further treatment may be needed to restore the natural acidity levels of the vagina. A more natural way is to build up your body's defences against thrush naturally by taking *Lactobacillus acidophilus* supplements (available from health shops) and eating two or three pots of live natural yogurt (which contains lactic bacteria) a day if you must take antibiotics.

The Contraceptive Pill

It has been suggested that the Pill could be a major cause of thrush in some women, for a number of reasons. First, because the Pill alters the body's natural hormonal balance to prevent ovulation. The combined pill releases synthetic progesterone and oestrogen, the female sex hormones, into the bloodstream in a similar way to the body during pregnancy.

The hormone changes that the Pill brings about can affect some women's sugar metabolism, encouraging thrush to grow, although the low dosage pills cause less metabolic change than the others. However, if you are taking the Pill your vaginal moisture and discharge can increase quite significantly, and this too can be a predisposing factor in encouraging the fungus to grow. Increased discharge can also set off vaginal infections.

The Pill can also make the vagina less acidic, and as we've seen, the yeast organism thrives in an alkaline environment. It can also upset our friendly intestinal flora, which are responsible for stopping the growth of the yeast. And long-term usage of oral contraceptive pills can eventually lead to deficiency in vitamin C and the B vitamins, among other nutrients, which can weaken the immune system and make the body more susceptible to thrush.

'I kept on getting thrush followed by cystitis, and I must have tried everything that was supposed to get rid of it. For three years it plagued me and then I had to come off the Pill for health reasons and I haven't had an attack since.'

MICHELLE, 28

IUDs

The inter-uterine device, or IUD, is a small flexible plastic or plastic and copper device which is inserted into the womb, and it's the second most popular method of contraception.

It works by preventing a fertilized egg from implanting in the womb, but it has its disadvantages – particularly if you are predisposed towards thrush. The chances of getting a pelvic infection are higher with an IUD than any other contraceptive methods, and so women who have had a history of pelvic infection should not have one fitted. IUDs can also activate old infections and cause bleeding between periods, which can set off thrush. Furthermore, the thread which hangs down into the vagina to tell you the device is in place can sometimes harbour bacteria which, again, can set off an infection. If you are prone to thrush it might be a good idea to switch to another form of contraception.

Diaphragms

Diaphragms, or dutch caps, are barrier methods of contraception – the diaphragm fits over the cervix to prevent the sperm from entering the womb. The diaphragm is a flexible rubber dome which, if it is to be effective, must be used with a spermicide.

Although it is not common, badly fitting diaphragms can cause abrasions of the vaginal wall, usually in the form of painful ulceration. Although infection at the time of intercourse is uncommon, probably because of the spermicide, vaginal abrasions can predispose a woman to thrush. Some women forget about removing their diaphragms, which can provoke an infection. The spermicide itself can, albeit rarely, cause an allergy in a few women and set up local inflammation.

Pregnancy

We are far more susceptible than normal to thrush during pregnancy because of the hormonal changes that occur in our bodies. The high levels of oestrogen produced means more vaginal sugar is secreted. The vaginal secretions can increase considerably, and the more copious the secretions, the greater the risk of an infection. The vagina also becomes more alkaline, so we could hardly provide a better environment in which thrush can flourish. No wonder thrush is a common affliction during pregnancy.

If you suffer from persistent thrush, it's a good idea to try and get it under control before you give birth. Some anti-fungals are not recommended during the first trimester, but most pregnant women don't want to take drugs of any sort during their pregnancy anyway. However, there are natural alternatives you can try and we will be looking at some of these in the second half of the book. If you're suffering from thrush when the baby is born, it can be born with thrush in its mouth or digestive tract. This is not dangerous, but obviously better avoided.

Thrush and Menstruation

Our menstrual cycle is controlled by a delicate balance of the sex hormones progesterone and oestrogen. If the tiniest imbalance occurs, the menstrual cycle can be thrown into disarray and symptoms ranging from heavy and uncontrolled bleeding to no bleeding at all can take place. If our oestrogen level is too high, the increased vaginal sugar this causes can lead to thrush. Thrush is common just before a period, because the blood creates the sort of warm alkaline environment in which the yeast can thrive.

The Menopause

The menopause usually occurs between the ages of 44 and 55, although it can begin earlier. The ovaries start secreting smaller amounts of the hormone oestrogen and the decrease in oestrogen means a decrease in the vaginal sugar. After a while, unless you're taking hormone replacement therapy, the yeast has nothing to sustain it, and thrush can't recur.

Hooray, hooray, I hear you cry. But while the menopause is

taking place you can still be prone to vaginal infections. The vaginal secretions start to decrease, so the vagina becomes less well-lubricated – and more easily irritated. The vaginal walls become thinner and less elastic, which can make sex uncomfortable.

Unlubricated sex is painful because the penis can cause abrasions, and when the skin is scratched or broken there's a very high chance that it can become infected. Using a water soluble lubricating jelly such as KY jelly (not Vaseline) can help. Hormone replacement therapy alleviates the problem of dryness, although it can also predispose you towards thrush because of the high levels of oestrogen.

Diabetes

Recurrent thrush is common among diabetic women who don't manage their diabetes efficiently. Diabetes affects sugar metabolism. Diabetics cannot store and utilize glucose properly, and unless they control the disease properly with insulin and diet they can lose sugar in their urine and have increased glucose vaginal secretions, which makes them very susceptible to thrush.

If the diabetes is controlled properly the urine should be free from sugar; a diet cutting out yeasts, yeast substances, cheeses, vinegar, alcohol, honey, oranges, and pickles also helps. If their male partner is diabetic, some women may have an increased risk of getting thrush.

Corticosteroids

These are used to treat such conditions as asthma, arthritis, acne and eczema, and are usually used as cream or inhaled. They work by suppressing the inflammatory reaction, so they relieve the symptoms rather than provide a cure. Since inflammation is our body's natural response to invading bacteria, this weakens the body's ability to fight off any threatened invasion of *candida*. Long-term use of inhaled steroids like becotide, which is prescribed for asthma, can cause thrush in the mouth.

Sex

Although thrush isn't really a sexually transmitted disease in the same way as gonorrhoea or trichomonas, as we have seen, your male partner can develop mild signs of a yeast infection. If he doesn't get it treated he'll keep on reinfecting you, so sex during a thrush attack isn't a great idea.

Apart from which, sex while you've got thrush can be mighty uncomfortable. All that friction against a tender and inflamed vagina and vulva can prevent healing, and semen can act as a good growth medium for thrush. It can take a long time to get rid of thrush if you don't refrain from sex during the healing period.

> 'All during my time at university I had recurring thrush. I would go off to an STD clinic and get pessaries and cream and it didn't occur to me at the time that my boyfriend might have something to do with it. In fact, he got quite sniffy when I suggested it. But after I broke up with him I never had another attack. I'm sure he had something to do with it.'
>
> SHEILA, 34

Your Immune System

Your general health is important in warding off recurrent attacks of thrush. If your general health is poor and your immune system becomes weakened, you will find it harder and harder to fight off attacks of thrush. Your immune system is undermined by many aspects of 20th-century living – stress, overwork, poor diet, pollution, artificial food additives, addictions, alcohol and smoking – to name but a few. All these factors sap your strength and put greater pressure on an already overloaded immune system, and make you more vulnerable to illness.

In chapter 7 we shall be looking at the immune system and how to strengthen it in more detail: meanwhile, the best way to build up your immune system is to eat a highly nutritional diet rich in fibre, fresh vegetables and fruit, ensure you get enough sleep and to manage your stress efficiently.

Cystitis

Cystitis and thrush very often go together: one seems to trigger off attacks of the other in susceptible women. Cystitis means a lot of things to a lot of people, but generally it's taken to mean inflammation of the bladder. It can be the bane of some women's lives as it can keep on recurring and, unlike thrush, the symptoms can sometimes be disabling.

As with thrush, the problem isn't helped by our poorly designed genital area. The urethra (the entrance of the tube that carries urine out of the bladder) and vagina share a common opening, and that opening is so close to the anus that the risk of infection from the anus is immense. Many infections are caused by bacteria from the lower bowel called *E. coli* (*Escherichia coli*), which will easily find its way from the bowel where it lives quite harmlessly, up the urethran tract and into the bladder where it is anything but harmless. Cystitis can also follow sex, giving rise to the epithet 'honeymoon disease'.

Cystitis can be a wretched, painful disease whose symptoms include pain on passing water – and sometimes you have to do so with such frequency that life has to be planned around the availability of toilets – and in severe cases, fever and backache. If it is not treated it can cause serious problems if it gets into the kidneys.

One reason why cystitis and thrush are such good friends is because doctors often prescribe antibiotics to treat cystitis, and as we've seen, antibiotics can harm your friendly intestinal flora and so trigger off an attack of thrush. If you must take antibiotics, take precautions against thrush such as lactobacilli supplements and two or three pots of live natural yogurt a day during the course. A good remedy you could obtain from a medical herbalist is couchgrass, which will not disturb your friendly flora. This is a diuretic, which will increase your urine output, but it also has anti-inflammatory and analgesic qualities, and is a natural antibiotic.

Many women who have had recurring cystitis have learned how to prevent it by carrying out a scrupulous hygiene ritual, which prevents the bacteria from finding its way to the urethra. This includes wiping the vagina or anus from front to back, rather than the other way round, washing yourself after using the lavatory and passing urine after sexual intercourse – essential, as sex can cause germs to get into the bladder. Angela Kilmartin, who has done much to help cystitis sufferers, gives a detailed account of how you can keep cystitis at bay in her book *Understanding Cystitis* (Century Arrow).

Stress

Holistic health practitioners and many orthodox medical practitioners are now seeing a link between stress and thrush.

Stress is not an illness. It's not even any one symptom, but a whole variety of symptoms which can be provoked in response to virtually any situation. It's not the stress that is a problem but our reaction to it, and how we handle it. It's our inability to handle stress, so that we react inappropriately to a situation, that can cause the physiological symptoms that can make stress a problem, weaken our immune system and leave us open to all manner of infections.

Stress triggers off increased amounts of adrenalin which can have an effect on our sex hormones, which in turn can lead to changes in the menstrual cycle and patterns, alter the balance in the vagina and precipitate an attack of thrush.

Continual stress pushes up our demand for nutrients, which can weaken the immune system and make us even more susceptible to thrush. If we learn how to manage our stress we can make it work for us in a positive way, and in chapter 6 we will look at various relaxation and stress management techniques. Better still, we should try and avoid stressful situations altogether, as far as is possible.

Damp Living Conditions

Some people find that they develop thrush when the weather is damp. Damp houses can also be responsible for recurrent thrush attacks: the yeast can even be stimulated by the sort of mildew or mould that's found on houseplants, outside walls, under sinks, behind toilets and baths, in cellars, in food cupboards or under carpets. Ensuring your house is dry and properly heated, and avoiding damp musty places, is sometimes enough to keep thrush from recurring.

Soaps, Bubble Baths and Deodorants

Highly perfumed soaps, talcum powder, vaginal deodorants or 'wipes', and bubble baths can aggravate thrush and trigger off attacks in susceptible women. They should be avoided. If you really must use soap, make sure it's completely natural and free of allergens like Simple soap, but it's better not to use soap on your genital area at all. Instead, wash with warm water using a shower spray, or moistened cotton wool. During a thrush attack, use cotton wool soaked in pharmaceutical olive oil.

Flannels can cause recurrences of thrush, unless they're boiled every day, as they can harbour bacteria. So can towels. It's better to pat your genital area dry with tissues if you haven't got a clean towel, and never share a towel. If you must add something to your bath, only use natural baby oil, and bear in mind that very hot baths can encourage the yeast organism to grow. If you are prone to thrush, bathe in warm water or shower.

Vaginal deodorants have, hopefully, gone out of fashion, although they seem to have been replaced by vaginal wipes – specially impregnated cleansing tissues with which to clean your genital area should you need to do so.

Products like these are usually completely unnecessary, expensive and encourage a false fastidiousness which can actually lead to thrush. They can kill off our natural lactobacilli and dry out our vaginas. Worst of all, they make us feel that vaginas are dirty, smelly parts of our bodies whereas the reverse is the case.

A woman's natural vaginal odour is not offensive – indeed, most men find it a turn-on. Why try and cover it up? Of course we should keep our genital area clean, but that's easily done with warm water or olive oil. Putting highly scented talcum powder on your outer genital area isn't a good idea either, for the powder can find its way into the vagina – and a link has been shown between talcum powder and ovarian cancer.[1]

Lack of Air

The *candida* organism thrives in a warm, dark, damp environment, so by wearing tight nylon underwear, jeans and leotards, you are providing it with the perfect place to grow.

Thrush cases soared after tights became more popular than stockings, and tight briefs replaced loose knickers. Wearing no knickers at all during a thrush attack will hasten its demise, and wearing loose cotton knickers the rest of the time will help ensure thrush doesn't recur. Stockings or crotchless tights instead of tights, and baggy trousers instead of jeans provide the sort of cool environment thrush hates.

Tampons

Tampons can have an aggravating effect if you suffer from thrush, particularly if you don't change them regularly, as they can cause ulcers in the vagina and set off an infection.

Diet

Yeast thrives on refined carbohydrates, so if your diet consists mainly of sugary, junk food with plenty of white bread, cakes, pastries and alcohol, you are making sure the yeast inside you is well-nourished.

Some women have noticed a link between a high sugar intake and thrush. Sometimes thrush can follow a candy binge, although one reason could be that many women get sugar cravings during their premenstrual period, and indulge in huge sweet-eating binges. But as we've seen, you can be vulnerable to thrush during the premenstrual period for other reasons, and perhaps that's the predisposing factor.

Whether or not there's a dietary connection, the fact is that a poor diet lacking in nutrients and high in sugar is certainly going to weaken your immune system, and make you susceptible to infections like thrush.

As you can see, there are many reasons why thrush can occur. Some are more important than others, but if you've been a persistent thrush sufferer, you will probably want to know about all the factors that can precipitate and aggravate thrush, no matter how trivial they might appear.

But thrush is only one of a whole list of genital infections, many of which share similar symptoms. In the following chapter we will be looking at what else it could be.

Chapter 3

WHAT ELSE COULD IT BE?

A S FAR AS SOME PARTS of the body are concerned, there are times when we women definitely get a raw deal. Not only do we we get lumbered with monthly periods for half our lives – and no matter how much some people bang on about periods being a wonderful celebration of our femininity, all the women I know think they're a pain – but we are wide open to a variety of problems which can affect our genital organs. In fact, some medical insurance companies charge women more than men for these reasons.

Most of these afflictions are trivial, and the symptoms little more than uncomfortable; some are not. So it pays to be aware of just what could go wrong.

The first time thrush strikes can be frightening, especially if we haven't a clue what's wrong. Ignorance makes us fear the worst. I once shared a flat with a girl who thought her first thrush attack was gonorrhoea, even though she was still a virgin. Because we equate our genital area with sex, it's hard to think of any problems 'down there' as being anything other than sex-related. So it's not surprising that the first thought that occurs to many women when they have any sort of genital disorder is venereal disease and the second is cervical cancer.

This isn't helped by the fact that the symptoms of thrush can be remarkably similar to many other common genital disorders. My doctor told me that the majority of women presenting themselves in his surgery complaining of thrush hadn't actually got it. Most had merely got a heavier than normal vaginal discharge for any number of reasons, but because they knew no better they automatically assumed the worst.

Vaginal infections invariably cause vaginal discharges – but not all discharges are as a result of infection. All women have a regular vaginal discharge – that's natural. Hopefully, most women know what is normal for them and don't confuse the normal occasions when their vaginal flow increases – two or three days before a period, at the time of ovulation, or when they are sexually aroused – with an infection. It's when there's some sort of change in your normal pattern of vaginal discharge that it's time to check that there's nothing amiss.

Women who have suffered one attack of thrush usually know how to recognize the symptoms if it recurs, and many don't bother to consult a doctor unless it persists, preferring to try self-help remedies. But thrush does sometimes accompany other vaginal infections, which is why you should always consult a doctor if you've never had thrush before and you've got a heavy discharge, particularly if it is an offensive colour and it smells. You should also always see a doctor if you're in pain or some discomfort, or if sex is painful, particularly if you think you may be at risk from venereal disease.

Even if you're an old hand at diagnosing thrush symptoms, you should always seek medical help if the symptoms persist. It's easy to mistake thrush for other complaints, and it's better to be safe than sorry. And it's useful to know what else it could be.

Trichomonas

Trichomonas (trich or TV) is a very common vaginal infection usually passed on through sexual contact, although it is not unknown for it to be picked up from damp towels and flannels. It's also possible for it to be passed on via a splash from an unflushed lavatory.

Sometimes an old infection can become active on its own for no apparent reason, and you are at your most susceptible just after a period. It is caused by a tiny parasite, *Trichomonas vaginalis*, which can live in the vagina, urethra, bladder and Bartholin's glands (see page 36), and the symptoms are very similar to thrush. It's probable that a lot of sexually active women are actually infected with trichomonas during their reproductive years and don't even realize they're infected because they show no symptoms.

Like thrush, trichomonas is characterized by a discharge, but this discharge is thin and yellowy-green and can smell quite dreadful. Other symptoms include severe itchiness in the vagina and around the perineum, vulval soreness, and a burning sensation rather like cystitis when you pass urine if the bladder becomes infected. The vagina can feel tender, and the vulva become swollen and inflamed. Pain during sex is often the reason which drives sufferers to seek treatment.

It's important not to have sex if you think you've got trichomonas until you're completely cured as you can infect your partner, although there is evidence that spermicides used with a diaphragm can protect against trich.[1] Then again, if you've got it badly, sex is probably the last thing on your mind.

A man can carry the organism but very often he won't show any symptoms, so if you're being treated for trichomonas it's important your partner gets treated too, or you'll go on passing it backwards and forwards *ad infinitum*.

If you think you've got trichomonas, you should go to your doctor or your local sexually transmitted disease clinic for treatment. The sexually transmitted disease clinic, or genito-urinary clinic as it tends to be known nowadays, is the best place to go as they have the facilities to test for it and treat you right away. If you don't, and the organism finds its way to your uterus and fallopian tubes, it could lead to a pelvic inflammatory infection which can block the tubes and lead to infertility.

A swab will probably be taken of the discharge for analysis and if it's found to be infected your doctor will probably prescribe metronidazole or nimorazole. Metronidazole is a strong antibiotic which can cause unpleasant side-effects. It should not be taken during pregnancy, or while breast-feeding, and the side effects include nausea, furred tongue with an unpleasant taste, urticaria rashes, depression, anorexia and, if you drink alcohol while you are taking it, severe vomiting.

Because it is an antibiotic you risk an attack of thrush if you take it. If you must take it, start preparing your defences: eat live yogurt several times a day, or take live *Lactobacillus acidophilus* supplements. These will help support the friendly bacteria which will be in danger of being wiped out by the antibiotics, and leave your body open to the thrush organism.

Another way to help ward off thrush while you are taking antibiotics is to put a peeled clove of garlic into your vagina. Garlic is a potent natural antibiotic: either wrap it in a piece of muslin with a piece of strong cotton thread tied to it so you can get it out easily, or thread a piece of cotton through the clove. Change the clove every four or five hours – but be prepared to smell like a French bistro!

Cervical Erosion

The cervix, or neck of the womb, connects the vagina with the womb. It is constantly secreting mucus, and the quantity and texture varies throughout the menstrual cycle according to the level of the sex hormones progesterone and oestrogen being produced at the time.

Sometimes a heavier than normal discharge can be due to a cervical erosion. This sounds a lot more alarming than it actually is: it's not the wearing away of tissue, but an inflamed patch on the cervix which occurs because the normal cervical tissue has been replaced by cells which usually lie in the cervical canal.

This can happen after or during pregnancy, or as a result of taking the contraceptive pill, because of the hormonal action, and the result is that the cervix produces a lot more mucus. The discharge that occurs when this happens can be bloody and therefore rather alarming, particularly if it occurs after sex, but it is harmless. However, the increased secretions make you more prone to infections, including thrush, so it might be an idea to take *acidophilus* supplements as we've just noted.

Cervical erosions are often picked up at routine examinations during pregnancy, or during a cervical smear, but if you have any sort of bloody discharge it's advisable to have a pelvic examination. Erosions usually clear up on their own, and a doctor will usually only suggest treatment if the symptoms persist. Treatment usually consists of cauterizing, or burning off the cells in the cervix with an electric or chemical cautery or a laser, a minor operation which can be done without an anaesthetic. Most erosions, however, present no symptoms and need no treatment.

Herpes

'O'er ladies' lips, who straight on kisses dream,
Which oft the angry Mab with blisters plagues'

Actually, the Bard was referring to Herpes simplex 1, or the cold sore virus, which puts in its unwelcome and ugly appearance on your lips when you've got a cold, or are run down. Genital herpes is usually caused by Herpes simplex 2, but either can cross over: from mouth to genitals during oral sex, or by inadvertently touching an infectious cold sore and then touching your genitals.

This most common virus infection was around long before *Romeo and Juliet* was written, and is usually passed on during sex. It can often be mistaken for thrush or even cystitis, as the characteristic painful blisters can be hidden behind the labia or are so small they can't be seen, so the only obvious symptoms are itching and sometimes a discharge. A bad attack can produce a fever, and after the blisters burst it can be very painful. You may also find it difficult to pass urine, which is why some people confuse it with cystitis.

Symptoms include first sores, then blisters. It is while the blisters are present that herpes is at its most infectious, and you must not have sex. Eventually the blisters burst and dry up, and the healing process is completed. Herpes causes a lot of distress because it can recur, and keep on recurring until the body can build up its defences against it.

There is nothing that can actually cure herpes, but an attack can be relieved by taking salt baths or bathing the area in a salt solution (about 1 teaspoon salt to a pint of warm water). Ice packs (crushed ice wrapped in a damp towel) relieve the pain, and a little witch hazel will help dry out the sores. As with thrush, keeping your genital area cool by avoiding tight nylon clothing helps.

Once you've got herpes you've got it for life, but it doesn't usually recur unless you're run down and your immune system is too weak to fight it off, so staying healthy and eating a well-balanced diet with plenty of fresh fruit, vegetables and wholefoods helps keep it at bay. Sometimes a recurrence can be triggered off by a vaginal infection, and stress plays a big part in triggering off herpes, so learn how to manage your stress by using relaxation techniques (see chapter 6).

There is a slight link between genital herpes and cervical cancer. If you suffer an attack of herpes, you should have cervical smears every year.

Vaginal Warts

These are painless but often itchy lumps of skin that can appear in the vagina, the vulva (the external genital area) or the perineum (the sensitive area between the anus and the vaginal opening) and are also caused by a virus. They may appear singly or in large groups, are usually small and pimply but can be uncomfortably large, and are most common in women between the ages of 25 and 35.

They are transmitted during sex, although if you've got warts on your hands you can pass them on if you touch your genital area. They don't usually appear until about three months after infection, and once they begin to grow they can spread; even more so if you're pregnant. They are harmless, but because there is a link between warts and cervical cancer, you should always see your doctor if they appear and have yearly smear tests. They can be painlessly burned off with lasers or chemical or electrical cautery.

Bartholin's Cysts or Abscesses

On either side of the vagina are the Bartholin's glands, tiny glands whose function is to secrete a mucus which keeps the vulva moist and healthy. Occasionally one of these glands can become infected and an abscess can form. It swells up and starts producing a profuse discharge, and it is unbelievably painful – and I speak as one who knows!

Passing urine makes the pain worse and the effect is not unlike peeing broken glass. An abscess will usually need lancing and draining by a doctor, although sometimes it can disappear of its own accord. The entrance to the gland can also get blocked up, causing a large cyst to appear: if a course of antibiotics doesn't shift it, a small operation might be needed to cut it out.

Pubic Lice, or Crabs

The pubic louse is a relative of the head louse, and although it is a tiny insect, it looks like a crab. The mere mention of pubic lice causes some people's scalp to crawl, let alone their pubic hair, but it's a very common parasite.

They're usually transmitted during sex, although they can be caught from infected bedding or towels. The louse gets into the pubic hair and sucks the blood from its unfortunate host, leaving a trail of itching spots in its wake. It lays eggs which hatch out and carry on biting, blood-sucking and laying eggs until, if left untreated, a veritable colony can be seen as tiny whitish specks.

The most usual symptom is itching, and you should seek medical help at a sexually transmitted disease clinic if you suspect you have lice, as it's possible you have another sexually transmitted disease as well. Crabs must be treated with malathion or carbaryl cream or lotion.

Chlamydia

Although it's only been recognized relatively recently, doctors believe that chlamydia has been around for a long time under a different name – NSU, or Non-Specific Urethritis.

Chlamydia is becoming the commonest sexually transmitted disease. It's caused by the bacterium *Chlamydia trachomatis*, and it can infect the vagina and the cervix. In men, a discharge from the penis generally follows infection by chlamydia, but some men may carry the organism and infect their sexual partners without being aware of it, because they have no symptoms. Many women also show no symptoms; some can have a dirty white frothy discharge, or feel sore around the vulva, or experience pain when they're passing urine. These appear around a fortnight after infection.

Because it is often symptomless, chlamydia is often only diagnosed when women present themselves for treatment for a different, often unrelated complaint. The sinister side of chlamydia is that if it's left untreated, it can lead to pelvic inflammatory disease, which can include infections of the fallopian tubes. When this happens, the tubes can become scarred or blocked, and so cause infertility. The chance of an ectopic pregnancy is high after PID.

If you have any reason for thinking you might be infected with chlamydia – if you've had sex with a partner you think might be infected, or if you're showing any symptoms you think might be chlamydia – go to an STD clinic as soon as you can, and take your partner with you. You are most at risk if you're young, and have a lot of sexual partners.

Chlamydia, like trichomonas, is treated with the antibiotic metronidazole, so guard yourself against an attack of thrush by eating large amounts of live yogurt at least four times a day, taking live supplements of acidophilus and garlic, and wearing loose cotton underwear.

Pelvic Inflammatory Disease

This is a general term to describe inflammation caused by infection of the uterus, cervix, fallopian tubes or ovaries. Sometimes it can be caused by an IUD, or diseases like gonorrhoea or chlamydia. It occasionally happens after an abortion, and very occasionally, after a burst appendix. It must be treated by a doctor without delay as it can lead to the development of abscesses on the uterus or tubes, and the resulting scar tissue can block the tubes, causing infertility.

Symptoms include a horrible-smelling vaginal discharge, fever, high temperature, pains in the back and tummy which are sometimes quite bad, menstrual cramps, tiredness, and painful intercourse. The only effective treatment is antibiotics – so, as before, mount your defences against a possible attack of thrush which could follow.

Bacterial Vaginosis (Non-Specific Vaginitis, Anaerobic Vaginitis)

This is one of the commonest causes of a vaginal discharge in sexually active women – the commonest in the United States. It is often confused with thrush or trichomonas as the symptoms are similar: it's very itchy and is accompanied by a profuse grey-white discharge which can smell ghastly.

The main organism implicated in bacterial vaginosis is *Gardnerella vaginalis*, and as it is thought to cause premature labour it is important to get treatment right away if you are pregnant. It seldom goes away spontaneously, although the symptoms usually disappear during a period, only to reappear when it is over.

As with trichomonas, the drug treatment is oral metronidazole, or local treatment with cream and pessaries. Metronidazole can, as we've seen, have unpleasant side-effects, but a recent study was performed[2] treating patients with metronidazole vaginal sponges, which worked well with no side-effects.

Non-Specific Genital Infections

As the name suggests, this means that the doctor can't actually identify what the organism is that's causing the symptoms – which are usually a vaginal discharge, pain on passing water and sometimes abdominal pain. Doctors will usually offer antibiotics at this point: you could try treating the infection by putting garlic into the vagina, as above, or taking garlic supplements, before you resign yourself to antibiotics.

Inflammation of the vagina can be caused by a forgotten

tampon. Forgetting tampons, particularly at the end of your period, is a common mistake and the results can be unpleasant: if it is left for more than a couple of days it can set off a nasty infection. The discharge which follows will be very unpleasant and smell horrible, and the tampon itself will probably be difficult to fish out.

Even if you are able to remove it yourself, see your doctor: forgotten tampons can cause toxic shock syndrome, a condition which can occur at menstruation when bacteria which are present in all of us start an infection in susceptible women. The bacteria can grow and overwhelm the vagina, and although the syndrome is very rare, it can be very dangerous. Keeping yourself in good health, changing tampons regularly, making sure you don't forget them and wearing towels when the flow is heavy or at night will help guard against this unpleasant but fortunately very rare complaint.

Vaginitis

Vaginitis is an irritation of the vagina and can usually be recognized by soreness, itching and dryness. After the menopause our levels of oestrogen, the female sex hormone, diminish. It's oestrogen which is responsible for the fluid which keeps the vaginal walls lubricated, and if the vaginal walls stop secreting this fluid, the vagina can become dry and inflamed, making sex uncomfortable and leaving us open to infection. Sex without lubrication, whether it is because you are not sufficiently aroused or because of vaginitis, can not only be painful: it can cause quite a lot of damage. Any tear in the vaginal wall leaves you wide open to infections, including thrush.

Although the symptoms of vaginitis include dryness and a scanty normal vaginal discharge, bleeding or blood-stained discharge might occur and that should always be checked out by a doctor. KY jelly, which can be bought from a chemist or drugstore, can help. If your vagina is inflamed after sex, bathe it in warm salt water – a teaspoon of salt to a pint of water.

Gonorrhoea

Gonorrhoea is the most common sexually transmitted disease. It's caused by bacteria which infect the opening of the urethra, the Bartholin's glands and the cervix, and it can spread into the uterus. You can only catch it by having sex with an infected partner, and sometimes the symptoms don't show in women until quite a time after infection – by which time they might have gone on unknowingly to infect other partners.

It's best to go straight to an STD clinic if you suspect you have gonorrhoea, as they have the facilities to test for it and treat it. If you don't treat it it can, like chlamydia, spread to the fallopian tubes and ovaries – and once that happens you run a high risk of becoming permanently sterile.

Most women see symptoms in their partners first: sores around the genitals and discharge from the penis are common. Women can also develop genital sores and a vaginal discharge, and experience pain and a burning sensation when they pass urine. Gonorrhoea can only be treated with antibiotics, so take anti-thrush precautions.

Cervical Cancer

Cervical cancer is the second most common cancer in women after breast cancer, and is most usually found in sexually active women. Symptoms can include an unpleasant vaginal discharge, bleeding between periods or after the menopause, but often there are no symptoms at all.

Yet cervical cancer is almost always entirely preventable: if all women had regular cervical smear tests they would be pinpointed as being susceptible to the disease long before it actually develops, as pre-cancerous cells can be identified and treated long before they turn into cancer. So it makes sense to have smears every three years, or every year if you're in an 'at risk' group – if you suffer from herpes, or have had genital warts. In the United States, all women over the age of sixteen are advised to have annual smear tests.

Smear tests are simple, painless and quick. Your doctor or family planning clinic can carry them out. Before taking the smear, the doctor will examine your vagina with a speculum, which is an instrument which separates the walls of the vagina so he or she can get a good look at the cervix and see whether or not it is inflamed.

The doctor will then rub a wooden spatula across the cervix to remove a smear of cells for analysis. It only takes a few minutes, and sounds far worse than it actually is. The smear will be sent off to a laboratory and the results should come through within a couple of weeks. If there is anything wrong, your doctor will contact you.

A smear test can also detect thrush, and the doctor will usually carry out a pelvic bi-manual examination at the same time. Don't be alarmed if you're told you need further investigations. It might be nothing. But even if pre-malignant cells are detected, they can be treated easily by removing the cells either with a laser or 'cone biopsy' – taking out a cone-shaped piece of tissue.

Cystitis

Cystitis and thrush often go together in a vicious circle of misery. To get an attack of cystitis just when you thought you'd got rid of your thrush can be really depressing. And like thrush, managing cystitis means changing your way of life.

Cystitis is an inflammation of the bladder, and is caused either by trauma – that is, bruising during sex – or infection, because of the poor design of the female body which means that the urethra, the outlet which takes the urine out of the body, is situated close to both the vaginal opening and the anus. This makes it relatively easy for bacteria to get into the urethra and set off an infection. If your vagina is irritated because of thrush, this can affect the urethra.

It can be ghastly, especially if it recurs frequently. Sufferers feel ill and feverish, and have frequent and urgent needs to pass urine which can be toe-curlingly painful if they actually manage it.

Cleanliness and good hygiene can help prevent cystitis.

Ensuring you wipe from front to back when you go to the lavatory helps stop bacteria from getting into the urethra. Unfortunately, bad attacks of cystitis tend to get treated with antibiotics which, of course, can trigger off an attack of thrush, which can cause cystitis . . .

So avoid antibiotics unless you're desperate. If you have to take them, go on an anti-thrush regime of live natural yogurt, garlic and live supplements of *acidophilus* as described earlier. Better, try and prevent cystitis from happening by taking the same sort of precautions you would against thrush (see chapter 12).

Avoid chemical irritation – don't use vaginal deodorants, bubble baths, strong soaps, or detergents. Wear cool, loose cotton underclothes. Cut sugar out of your diet. Drink lots of water. Pass urine before and after sex and keep scrupulously clean. Hopefully, that will prevent the infection from starting.

Now we've seen what else your symptoms could be, in the next chapter we'll look at what treatment is available if you seek medical help.

Chapter 4

WHAT DOCTORS CAN DO

Y OUR FIRST ATTACK of thrush can be emotionally and physically devastating. It's worrying because you probably don't know what it is. It makes you feel unclean, and it doesn't do a lot for your sex life, either. It's somehow a little difficult to summon up a grand passion when you itch like mad and are emitting a profuse and unpleasant discharge.

Those unfortunate enough to suffer from recurrent thrush can usually tell when an attack is imminent, and prepare themselves accordingly. Often, they don't bother to see a doctor, other than perhaps to collect a prescription to treat the symptoms. The thought of maybe having to have an internal examination is enough to deter the hardiest soul.

We've seen that you can try and stop thrush from developing by taking live *acidophilus* supplements, eating live natural yogurt three or four times a day, inserting garlic into the vagina or taking garlic supplements (see page 34). You can also try putting a teaspoon of yogurt directly into your vagina each night for a week, either using an applicator, or putting it on the end of a tampon. You can try bathing in a vinegar solution – one teaspoon vinegar to a pint of lukewarm water, or just sitting in a bowl full of vinegar and water to help acidify the vagina.

If the symptoms persist, particularly if you've recently changed your sexual partner, you must see a doctor.

Always see a doctor if your discharge is different from usual, if it is very heavy, offensive (i.e. smelly and a horrible colour), if you've got any sort of genital swelling, or if you're in pain, particularly when you have sex. You might think it's thrush but you can't be absolutely sure without proper tests and a medical examination. For as we've seen in the previous chapter, thrush not only goes hand in hand with many other vaginal infections, it can also have similar symptoms. And some infections must be treated by a doctor.

Going to a doctor when you've got a genital complaint is never much fun. Who enjoys talking about the malfunctioning of their most intimate organs? Who looks forward to being examined by a sometimes less than sensitive doctor?

It's not surprising that some women are nervous about seeking medical treatment for genital complaints. You can't blame them. Most doctors are men and some are not particularly sympathetic when it comes to gynaecological problems. By and large, they can't understand why many women find it acutely embarrassing to have the most private parts of their bodies, which are usually reserved for their lovers, come under scrutiny. And at the end of the day, no male doctor can really understand what it's like to have uniquely female genital disorders because he is unable to experience them himself. So it can be hard trying to explain to some macho doctors why thrush is making you so depressed, even though it's a relatively minor complaint.

If you can't bring yourself to see your usual male doctor, you can ask to see a female doctor. Group medical practices are the norm nowadays, and nearly all surgeries have a female doctor attached to them; even if you are registered with a male doctor you are entitled to see another doctor within the same practice. If there is no woman doctor there might be a practice nurse who can take swabs.

In the UK, most big towns and doctors surgeries have well woman clinics which deal specifically with women's problems. These are usually staffed by experienced nurses, female gynaecologists or sympathetic males. NHS well woman clinics are, of course, free but there are also 'charity' clinics which make a small charge for a consultation and examination, and private clinics which sometimes make a large charge for the same thing. So check the cost before you make an appointment.

Some women prefer to go to private clinics because they cannot face going to see their family doctor about a problem like thrush, especially if they know them well. They wrongly see thrush as a sexually transmitted disease and feel embarrassed and ashamed about having it. Some don't even realize it *is* thrush if they've never had it before, and are convinced they've got some sort of venereal disease. They prefer to see an anonymous doctor because they know they will never have to see them again.

It's hard to cope with these sort of feelings. They arise from the feelings of guilt most women have instilled into them at an early age, and the fact that many mothers bring their daughters up to deny their sexuality and believe that their genitals are dirty and somehow shameful. It is difficult not to equate our genitals with sex: they are an intimate, private part of our body that we only want to share with chosen partners, not a strange male doctor. It can be difficult understanding that a genital disorder is exactly the same as any other disorder: after all, thrush also affects the mouth and nobody has any qualms about seeing a doctor for that.

'I was a student when I got my first attack of thrush and I had no idea what it was. It coincided with my first sexual relationship, and I'd done a lot of soul-searching before I slept with this boy. When the thrush appeared, I thought it was some sort of divine judgement. I would rather have died than go to our doctor, who was a friend of my father's, and I was convinced it was VD. Thank heavens I saw an ad at college for an STD clinic. They were so nice there – and most important, they made me realize I wasn't alone, that it was a really common complaint.'

SARAH, 38

Whichever doctor you opt for, he or she will almost certainly give you a pelvic examination, particularly if it's the first time you've presented yourself with the symptoms. It is useful if you know the date of your last period, so the doctor knows at what stage of your menstrual cycle you are at, as the state of your vaginal and cervical secretions changes throughout the cycle. It must drive doctors mad when they see a constant stream of women who haven't got a clue when their last period occurred.

It's not painful, or even really uncomfortable, but it's unrealistic to pretend that a pelvic examination is a load of laughs. However, relaxing and not resisting makes the experience a lot more bearable, as does a sensitive, gentle doctor (preferably one who's warmed his or her hands first!). When you are tense, and your muscles are fighting against it, a pelvic examination can be very uncomfortable indeed.

The doctor will probably do a bi-manual examination. You lie on your back with your legs bent open (although some doctors prefer it if you lie on your side) while the doctor examines your vagina by putting two or three gloved fingers of one hand into the vagina while pressing down on your abdomen with the other. This helps the doctor to feel the shape and size of the uterus. He or she will then look for any lumps, swellings or abrasions on the vulva, and then gently insert a narrow metal or plastic instrument called a speculum into the vagina. As the vaginal walls are like soft collapsible folds, in order to get a good view of the vagina and cervix these folds have to be held aside. Once the speculum is in place, the doctor can fix its blades open, and this holds the walls open so he or she can see what sort of state the vagina and cervix are in.

The doctor will look for discharge, inflammation of the vaginal walls, abnormal discharge from the cervix, inflammation of the cervix, abrasions, signs of infection, damage or growths. He or she might take a swab of any discharge or perform a cervical smear test. (See page 42 for an explanation of the smear test.)

Although this is usually performed to detect pre-cancerous cells, it's a routine screening procedure and one that all women should have at least every three years: ideally, every year. Some doctor also use it for other diseases like thrush or trichomonas, while others don't like doing smears while thrush is present, as sometimes the yeast can cause abnormalities to appear which disappear as soon as the infection has gone.

STD Clinics

There is another way you can have thrush treated, anonymously and with complete confidentiality, and that's at your local sexually transmitted diseases clinic (STD), or genito-urinary clinic as they are often called nowadays.

STD clinics have come a long way since the dark days of the 'special' or venereal disease clinics that used to be advertised in public lavatories. They were almost always situated in the depths of the hospital and were usually decorated in as unappealing a way as possible, compounding the feeling of shame many of their patients felt when they turned up there for treatment. There's still an antipathy towards them from some women who feel embarrassed and ashamed at the very thought of seeking help from such a place.

This is a shame, because nowadays things have changed radically. STD clinics are usually situated in the main part of the hospital, and tend to be light, airy and pleasant places. The staff are friendly, sympathetic and understanding and, most important, highly experienced in treating not just sexually transmitted diseases, but all infections of the genito-urinary tract. The clinic is equipped with up-to-date diagnostic equipment, and tests can usually be carried out straightaway. Although thrush isn't strictly speaking a sexually transmitted disease, nevertheless, in 1987 over 50,000 women were treated for thrush at these clinics in Britain.

Probably the most attractive aspect about STD clinics is that you can quite literally walk in off the street and not even have to give your name to the staff there if you don't want to. Often you don't even need an appointment. The clinics operate a strict code of confidentiality, and won't contact your doctor if you don't want them to, nor do you need a doctor's referral to attend one. Furthermore, they usually go out of their way to be helpful and obliging, because if you have got a serious sexually transmitted disease they are anxious that you will co-operate about treatment, and not pass on the disease. They are the best places you could possibly go to for the treatment of genital infections.

If you want to see a woman doctor, most clinics will be happy to arrange for you to see one, even if there isn't one on duty at the time. Your local hospital, doctor or family planning clinic will give you the telephone number of your nearest STD clinic, or it might be listed in the telephone directory under sexually transmitted diseases. They usually have their own telephone line, which is quite separate from the main hospital switchboard.

At the clinic the doctor will ask you a lot of questions, some of which you may find embarrassing as they concern your sex life, but it is necessary to make a diagnosis. Then vaginal and cervical swabs will be taken, a cervical smear, a blood test, a urine test, and a chlamydia test. Then follows a bimanual pelvic examination. Your urine might be checked for sugar, as, although it is rare, you could be suffering from diabetes or hypoglycaemia if you have recurrent thrush problems.

A new accurate diagnostic test for thrush can produce results within minutes. The basis of the test is antibody-antigen agglutination reaction, and it has a sensitivity almost twice that of microscopy. Vaginal swabs are taken as normal and a drop is put on to a card slide which has been coated with antibodies to *candida*. If agglutination – or the clumping together of cells – takes place, the test is positive. Cultures might also be grown, however, to make absolutely sure, and you won't know the results of those for two days. Not until thrush or any other infection which might be present has been diagnosed will a doctor decide on treatment.

Sometimes it can be difficult to diagnose recurrent thrush, because cultures for *candida* from vaginal swabs are often negative when the disease is recurrent. This is because unless you are in the middle of a very severe attack, the organism is only present in small quantities and you may well have recently used an antifungal product. Doctors, therefore, often look as closely at your history as at the laboratory results.

What's On Offer?

If your doctor diagnoses thrush, he or she will probably prescribe anti-fungals in the form of creams, pessaries and gels, or antibiotics.

Anti-fungals reduce the yeast without killing it completely, to help your body restore its natural, healthy defences. The trouble with anti-fungals is that they can efficiently clear up an attack but they won't prevent a recurrence. They don't actually get to the root of the problem, and as thrush is often associated with a weak immune system, an acid-alkaline imbalance in the vagina or insufficient friendly bacterial flora, there's little point in treating the symptoms without looking for the underlying cause as otherwise it almost certainly will recur.

More about that later, but it's worth bearing in mind that drugs are no substitute for enhanced health. Although anti-fungals can save a lot of misery as they quickly clear up the symptoms, they're really only providing symptomatic relief, and the underlying cause could well mean thrush returns to haunt you.

Nystatin is a commonly prescribed anti-fungal drug which can be used as a cream, gel, pessaries, dusting powder or tablets (which are normally only used when thrush is very severe, or present in the mouth or gut). Names under which it is marketed are Nystan, Dermovate-NN; Gregoderm; Multilind; Nystaform; Nystan-Dome; Nystavescent; Tinaderm-M.

> 'It used to drive me mad – I used to get an attack of thrush and I'd go and get some pessaries from the doctor and it would clear up and then about a couple of months later back it would come. A friend told me about yogurt so the next time I had an attack I used anti-fungals and also ate loads of live yogurt. This seems to have stopped the thrush recurring.'
>
> BRYONY, 29

Other anti-fungals your doctor could prescribe include:

Econazole (which is marketed under the names Ecostatin, Gyno-Pevaryl, Peveryl), a broad spectrum anti-fungal agent which comes in the forms of cream, ointment and pessaries. It's not advised during early pregnancy, and can occasionally cause local skin irritation.

Clotrimazole (Canesten), an anti-fungal drug used in topical application which comes in the form of pessaries, cream and lotion. Very rarely it can cause sensitivity reactions of burning or irritation.

Femstat is an anti-fungal vaginal cream derived from butoconizole, which has recently been approved in the US and has fewer side-effects than others.

Miconazole (Monistat, Gyno-Daktarin), which comes as pessaries, coated tampons, cream or gel, and also in tablet form for treating oral thrush or for *candida* infections of the gut. Side-effects are rare but can include skin irritation, nausea and vomiting, and treatment should be continued for at least a week after the symptoms have gone.

Pessaries are usually prescribed for vaginal thrush. They're cone-shaped dissolving tablets which you should push up into the vagina as far up as possible. Don't worry about doing yourself harm – they're quite safe. There's no way you can push them into your uterus. Pessaries are often supplied with a plastic applicator, but a lot of women find it easier to use their fingers.

If the infection is confined to the vulva you might only be prescribed a cream to spread over the vulval area, but often both cream and pessaries are prescribed as they're the most effective. The pessaries should usually be inserted at night, but if you do have to wear them during the day, wear pads to prevent your underwear from staining. Some brands of pessaries can damage the rubber of diaphragms and sheaths, so check with your doctor if you use barrier contraception, and ask him for pessaries which don't.

How long the treatment lasts depends on which type of pessary you're prescribed and whether or not you get recurrent attacks. Some patients are given a supply of antifungal pessaries to use as and when they are required – that is, when the symptoms of thrush first appear. Some are given high doses of pessaries to use over six weeks, together with tablets to be taken by mouth. Others who suffer from severe recurrent thrush could be put on a long-term management regime which can last as long as a year. Oral anti-fungals are usually taken when the attack is severe, to prevent reinfection from the intestine, and some of these can make you feel sick. You must carry on taking them until your course of treatment has finished even if the symptoms have gone, otherwise the thrush will recur.

It's a good idea to treat your partner with anti-fungal cream, as well, even if he's not showing any symptoms.

If you're using vaginal pessaries you can help restore the natural acidity of your vagina by bathing it in a solution of vinegar and cold water (one teaspoon vinegar to a pint of water), or putting a menstrual sponge (a sponge which you use instead of tampons or towels) soaked in a vinegar solution into your vagina.

If you suffer from thrush and cystitis together, you may be prescribed antibiotics, but doctors are often loath to prescribe antibiotics for thrush because they know they can exacerbate the very problem the antibiotics are there to treat. Antibiotics, which is a loose title for any drug which is used to treat bacterial infections, should only be prescribed for thrush sufferers as a last resort as they can't discriminate in the bacteria they kill: as well as the harmful bacteria, they will also kill off any friendly vaginal flora, and that will leave you wide open to another attack of thrush.

However, occasionally there's no other way, particularly if you are a frequent cystitis sufferer, and so during the course of treatment you should take precautions against an attack of thrush as described previously.

The newest and most effective drug used to treat thrush is an antibiotic called fluconazole. This potent drug is only usually prescribed when all else fails. It only needs to be taken in a single dose, and can eliminate *candida* from both the vagina and rectal area, and it's looked upon as a major advance in the symptomatic treatment of thrush. It's expensive, which is why it's unlikely to become widely available, and it hasn't yet been pronounced safe to be taken during pregnancy, or by those with kidney disease. Its side-effects include nausea, abdominal discomfort and headaches, but because it is still relatively new doctors only prescribe it in very severe cases of thrush.

One of the few over-the-counter preparations you can buy to treat thrush is Aci-Jel. This is a vaginal antiseptic jelly which, if used together with anti-fungals or antibiotics, can help restore acidity to the vagina. It's useful for most vaginal infections, and as its active constituent is acetic acid, the same as vinegar, it has the same antibacterial activity. But you'll probably get the same effect bathing in a vinegar solution – and it's cheaper. Nappy rash cream is good for relieving soreness in the vulval area, as is witch hazel.

These are the orthodox ways of treating thrush, and initially, they are usually beneficial. But like all forms of orthodox medicine, treating thrush in this way will stop the symptoms without getting to the root cause. Many women who have been treated only with anti-fungals report frequent recurrences of their thrush. Yet thrush is a condition which can be contained, by keeping the body as healthy as possible by following a highly nutritious diet, managing stress efficiently, and by taking anti-thrush precautions when you are at risk. Orthodox and complementary medicine can work together very efficiently to combat thrush.

In the following chapters, we shall be looking at various ways of achieving a state of optimum health – naturally. Not every therapy will be suitable for every person. It's up to you to find the one that suits you best, the one that you think will help you to remain in the best of health. Because that's the best way of ensuring thrush doesn't return.

Chapter 5

NATURALLY GOOD HEALTH

M ANY OF US are becoming disillusioned with orthodox medicine. Overcrowded doctors' waiting rooms, unhelpful and overworked doctors, and drugs whose side-effects can be worse than the complaint for which they have been prescribed, have all helped to popularize alternative, or complementary medicine.

For whatever else it is, complementary medicine is safe. Whereas some new 'wonder' drug which has, its manufacturers claim, been thoroughly researched and tested, might have long-term effects which are not yet known about, no such risks exist with natural remedies, as most of them have been in existence for thousands of years.

But still many of us have come to see drugs as a cure-all, and we feel deprived if we leave a doctor's surgery without a prescription. If we have a sore throat, we ask for antibiotics. If we have a cold we take cold suppressants. If we have a cough, we take expectorants. Too impatient to put up with the irritating symptoms as the disease runs its course, often we try and suppress those symptoms, and as soon as they're gone we think we're better. Often we're not. We've just bought a bit more time until the next complaint comes along.

Even the mildest drugs can have side-effects, and some side-effects can be positively dangerous. People can have life-threatening allergies to penicillin. Antihistamines make you drowsy. Hormones can masculinize you. Some anti-fungal drugs can occasionally impair your liver function.

Fortunately, the wind of change is blowing through many of the more progressive doctors' surgeries, and more and more are resisting the urge to reach for their prescription pad as soon as a patient walks through the door. The emphasis is being laid on prevention.

Of course many drugs work. They save lives. And complementary medicine won't help much if you've got an appendix which is just about to rupture. But it's at least debatable that if you follow a healthy way of life in every respect, you might reduce your chances of ever needing surgery at all.

The holistic approach to medicine involves looking at the whole person, not just the symptoms; seeing each person as an individual. For although curing the symptoms might be convenient in the short term, it's not a long-term solution because you haven't got to the root of the problem. Many women find that although using anti-fungals brings almost immediate relief from thrush because it clears up the annoying discharge and stops the itching, it doesn't prevent thrush from recurring. And that's because symptomatic medicine doesn't find out why thrush occurred in the first place.

Holistic medicine is based on the belief that the body, mind, emotions and spirit must be absolutely balanced and in perfect harmony to keep in good health. In order to keep this balance, factors like our environment, family, relationships, even the food we eat are important – in other words, our way of life, which can either predispose us towards illness or help prevent it.

Holistic practitioners don't just see a body with certain symptoms: they work on the principle that everyone is an individual, and so everyone's needs are different. So the first consultation with a complementary medical practitioner will invariably consist of a long and detailed interview. Just as important is the part we can play in healing ourself: our attitude, our state of mind and our approach to life all play a part. It's now generally accepted that there's a link between cancer – and a whole lot of other illnesses, including thrush – and stress.

A measure of how widely accepted holistic medicine has become is that most large towns now have a natural health centre where it is possible to consult a wide range of even the most esoteric natural practitioners. Twenty years ago such a thing would not have been possible: then, even going to an osteopath – long regarded as the most 'acceptable' alternative practitioner – raised eyebrows.

Now, even the orthodox medical profession is starting to accept some of the better-known forms of natural medicine like acupuncture, osteopathy and homoeopathy, and has expressed an interest in trying to work together with its alternative counterparts. The British Royal Family, who have long been disciples of homoeopathy, must take some of the credit for helping homoeopathy to become recognized as the effective form of medicine it is.

There are many different forms of complementary medicine and many of them can be used for symptomatic relief, but if you visit a practitioner, he or she will do more than just dish out a herbal remedy or suggest a new diet. The practitioner will try and understand you and then prescribe for you as a whole person, as well as trying to discover the cause of any imbalances.

Complementary medical practitioners also take an interest in all aspects of their patients and their lives, to the extent that you may find some of the questions they ask puzzling and irrelevant, especially if you are used to a doctor who just reaches for his prescription pad as soon as you walk into the surgery. They have to ask them in order to build up a complete picture of you, a unique human being. They don't just see the part of you that needs treatment.

That is not to say that orthodox doctors don't see their patients as people. Some of them are terrific, and often realize that a woman who comes in ostensibly for one ailment is really seeking help for another. But many doctors are so overworked they simply haven't the time to give their patients the attention they often need, and because they are aware of this, a lot of women have difficulty talking to their doctors. Also, although the situation is improving, doctors traditionally have usually been white, male and middle class – difficult to relate to if you're from a different ethnic or social group. In a busy urban practice it might be difficult to see the same doctor twice, and so it can be impossible to build up any sort of close relationship with your doctor.

But sometimes doctors can become so blinkered in their quest to find a cure that they can forget that their patient is a human being, and only see them as an interesting case. Once, I was treated in hospital by a very well-known gynaecologist. He was a brilliant doctor, but he was awkward and uncomfortable talking to his patients, as was apparent when he went through an identical line of chat to each one. The only time he was really relaxed and natural was when he was discussing his patients' ailments in incomprehensible medical terms over their heads with his registrar. He found it difficult to see his patients as anything other than wombs – the complete opposite of an alternative medicine practitioner.

Thrush, to an alternative practitioner, is a symptom that all is not well with your whole way of life. Your body's harmony is upset, and until you can correct that harmony you can suppress the symptoms as often as you like but the thrush can still recur at any time. If thrush occurred in the first place because antibiotics have destroyed the friendly bacteria as well as the unfriendly bacteria in your body, unless you restore that bacterial balance, back it will come. If you suffer greatly from stress, you must understand that stress is damaging your life, triggering off attacks of thrush and other illnesses, and you must start to manage your stress; otherwise the thrush will just come back. If you developed thrush due to an immune system that has been weakened because you exist on a junk food diet, backed up by alcohol and cigarettes, and you cure the symptoms without changing your lifestyle as well, back it will come.

There is little point in only curing the symptoms if you persist in carrying on with a stressful, destructive lifestyle. Far better to try and get the balance right. You can't expect an orthodox symptomatic approach from a holistic practitioner: it's no good taking natural remedies and expecting them to cure your thrush if you're weakening your immune system by drinking to excess and smoking.

The upsurge in popularity that natural medicine is currently enjoying is part of the growing awareness many people have about their environment, as they realize that the lifestyle they have become used to cannot be sustained. The trend is towards natural foods and natural products. There's also a growing feeling that using animals on which to test potent and often dangerous drugs is not only offensive, it's not even always effective. Thalidomide was thoroughly tested on animals, but still proved to have terrible side-effects when used by women.

In the following chapters we shall be looking at the holistic approach to treating thrush – that is, treating the whole person as an individual, not just the symptoms. That's all very well, I hear you cry, but here am I being driven up the wall with itching and all I want is symptomatic relief – now!

Obviously, the holistic approach takes time. Rebuilding your dwindling stores of intestinal flora, or strengthening your immune system, or rebalancing your bodily harmonies isn't going to happen overnight. Here are some self-help remedies you can try if you want symptomatic relief without anti-fungals. Like all natural remedies, they work for some people and not for others. But they can't hurt you – and they might just do some good.

Stopping the Itching

Yogurt, as you will see, is mentioned throughout this book. That's because it has been acknowledged for a long time as one of the most useful natural remedies. Of course it goes without saying that the yogurt is live, natural and without added honey, fruit, sugar or anything else you can think of!

Yogurt can be soothing put into the vagina each night during an attack – about a teaspoonful either on a tampon or using an applicator or syringe, although it's messy. Yogurt also acidifies the vagina, and thrush hates acid. Not only that, but live yogurt contains the friendly flora *Lactobacilli* which help fight off the dreaded yeast, which is why naturopaths recommend eating two or three pots of yogurt a day during an attack.

Instant relief from itching can be obtained by putting an ice pack – that is, ice cubes wrapped in a cloth – onto the offending part, and sponging it with vinegar diluted in slightly warm water is soothing. Using one teaspoon of vinegar per pint of water, you can either soak a menstrual sponge in it and put it into your vagina, add a tablespoonful to your bath water or sit in a bowlful for twenty minutes (a tablespoonful to a large bowl of water). Some women like to douche with a vinegar solution, but douching must be done with care (see page 115), and not immediately before, during or after a period, or during pregnancy. Warm salt baths are soothing, and heal inflamed tissues, as does cotton wool soaked in witch hazel.

Garlic

Garlic is a wonderful natural antiseptic and promotes healing. Thread a length of cotton thread or dental floss through a garlic clove (it makes it easier to remove) and put it into your vagina. You can also wrap it in a piece of gauze or muslin if you prefer. Some people swear by nicking the garlic with a knife to allow the oil to seep out, others find this can be irritating. Experiment to discover what is best for you.

Leave the garlic overnight and then replace with a new clove. The only disadvantage about this is that you positively reek of garlic the entire time. Happily, though, odourless garlic supplements can now be bought and taking these every day can keep infection at bay and inhibit the growth of yeast. If you don't care about the smell, the best way of consuming garlic is fresh with meals. A clove chopped up in salad dressing is delicious.

Olive Oil

Virgin olive oil contains a substance called oleic acid which, taken daily, prevents the transformation of the yeast into its destructive fungal form. The most palatable way of taking it is probably in a salad dressing: frying it just will not do! The B vitamin biotin acts upon the yeast in a similar way.

Natural medicine and a whole new and healthy way of life can help keep you in the best of health without resorting to drugs. In the next five chapters we will be looking at how effective stress management, strengthening the immune system, herbal medicine, acupuncture and the right sort of diet can help keep thrush at bay – for good.

Chapter 6

HOW TO HANDLE STRESS

I F THERE'S ONE THING doctors and complementary medical practitioners tend to agree on, it's that there is a link between stress and many different illnesses, including thrush. It's even acknowledged that cancer can be triggered off as a result of a stressful lifestyle, and a lot of attention is being paid to anti-stress techniques.

Thrush is a complaint associated with lowered resistance, in which stress can play a major part. Thrush and stress can be a vicious circle which is hard to break. Stress can bring on an attack of thrush which in turn can create more stress, which can trigger off another attack of thrush, and so on. It can carry on like that until you can get your stress under control.

Stress is not in itself an ailment – it's doubtful if we could function properly as human beings without a modicum of stress. If we eradicated stress from our lives altogether, we'd probably be like zombies. Indeed, the sort of people who like spending their leisure hours jumping out of airplanes, climbing mountains or hang gliding derive a positive buzz out of the stress that flirting with danger inevitably brings. Stress is not the problem. It's how we handle it that's important.

Stress is all things to all people. It is really our reaction to any situation we might be faced with each day. Fear of the future. Of being made redundant. Of a marriage breaking down. Of illness.

Of failing exams. Some people can even find everyday tasks like cooking highly stressful if there is a deeper, underlying cause of stress in their lives to which they have not faced up. Stress is something we encounter all day, every day, but it's our response to it that causes problems.

What is stressful to one person might not be stressful to another: the same event might affect two people completely differently. One woman might sit in a traffic jam, deaf to the cries of the children moaning about how late they're going to be getting to school, because she is able to stay calm, switch her mind off and not let the potential stress in that situation overwhelm her.

Another woman might sit in the car drumming her fingers on the steering wheel, hooting the horn in anger and frustration, screaming at the recalcitrant children in the back and working herself up into a highly stressful state. She has allowed the stress in that situation to take her over.

Similarly, one person may find the strain of reaching the top at work stressful while another thrives on it, and couldn't envisage not working a sixteen-hour day. It all depends on whether or not you have a positive attitude towards life. Nervous breakdowns don't tend to happen to positive people.

Of course everybody will experience crises at some point in their lives with which even the most equable people will find hard to cope – divorce, death of a loved one, moving house or redundancy. Obviously, those sort of events are going to trigger off typical stress responses. It's completely normal to react to crises in that way. It's when your body fails to return to normal afterwards, when it starts reacting to everyday events in a stressful way so that eventually, the stress responses become the norm – that's when stress starts having a destructive effect.

If we handle potentially stressful situations in a positive way, stress can be made to work for and not against us – how else do you think high achievers get to the top? But if you handle stress in a negative way, your body becomes run down, and your immune system weak and unable to fight off infection, until your resistance becomes so low you become prey to a variety of illnesses – including thrush.

Stress allowed to run riot can overwhelm us, until its symptoms are with us the whole time. Soon, there's no respite: it eats away at us day in, day out, and the greater hold it exerts on us, the more damaging are its effects on our bodies. It pushes up our need for nutrients, and it can weaken the immune system, which can leave us wide open to a whole variety of illnesses, both physiological as well as psychological.

Fight or Flight

We have an innate response to stress which dates back to less complicated times, when there were only two choices available to us when we found ourselves in a potentially dangerous situation – fight or flight. This instinctive fight or flight mechanism protected our primitive ancestors when they were faced with a life-threatening situation: their response was either to fight the attacker, or to run away from it. To do neither probably would have meant they would be killed and so ultimately, the survival of the species depended on this response.

The body prepares for action, whether it is for fighting or running away, in a number of physiological ways. When the brain is alerted by fear, the adrenal glands produce a hormone called adrenalin, or epinephrine, which flows through the body and has a number of effects. It causes the muscles to tense in preparation for either fighting or running away, which is why we often feel trembling and aching when we're under stress.

It makes the blood vessels to the muscles relax so that more blood can be pumped to them to fuel all this extra work they are going to have to do. To compensate, other blood vessels contract, causing some parts of the body to be temporarily short of blood. That's why people under great stress or in shock look pale.

All this extra blood being pumped causes the heart to beat faster and the blood pressure to rise, which is why we can often feel a throbbing sensation in the neck and head. Extra work needs extra fuel: more oxygen is needed, so we start to breathe more quickly and more shallowly. The high levels of adrenalin coursing through us can cause stomach cramps, diarrhoea and nausea. Adrenalin

65

also affects the body's balance of water, which is why our mouths go dry and our skin starts to sweat. By now, we're poised and ready to fight or run away.

The trouble is, these responses aren't usually appropriate in today's world. They might be appropriate if you're faced with a mugger in an alleyway late at night, because that is a dangerous situation and your survival might depend on your response to it. But when you're experiencing these sort of reactions day in, day out, in response to situations like sitting in a traffic jam, or when the kids start playing up, or you have an argument with your husband, or when the dinner's spoilt, they're definitely not appropriate.

Nevertheless, many people do respond to seemingly trivial, everyday occurrences in this way, and it's their inability to respond appropriately which, if it goes on for a long period of time, can lead to ill-health. The only way to deal with stress problems is to learn how to discharge the body's stress response, whether it's by dealing with the problem that is causing the stress, or by minimizing its effect by learning anti-stress and relaxation techniques. Being able to relax will help you bring about a change in the way you respond to potentially stressful situations.

Our response to a threat or potentially stressful situation depends on our attitude towards it. How many times have you had a row with someone and let it prey on your mind all day? The more you think about it, the more you work yourself up, so that when you next meet the person you're so tense and wound up you feel like physically attacking them.

That's a negative way of dealing with a situation. A change of attitude and a more appropriate response in the aftermath of a row is to shrug your shoulders and make it up. Sure, it's hard to do. Our response to potentially stressful situations is deep-rooted, and the causes varied. How your parents reacted to stressful situations has a lot to do with how you react. If you had nervous parents who suffered from stress, the chances are you will, too. The experiences that have helped shape your life, and your environment, have a lot to do with it as well. It's difficult not to let stress overcome you if your partner's left you and you're living in a damp, one-bedroomed flat with a couple of kids and no income.

But attitudes can be changed, and the effects of stress can be lessened, and that's what we'll be looking at in the rest of this chapter.

> 'I kept getting thrush when I was at college, over and over again. It wasn't until I compared notes with a friend of mine that I realized my thrush always recurred during the run up to my exams when I felt at my most stressful.'
>
> STEFIE, 26

It's important to recognize the early signs of stress: irritability, over-reacting to trivial incidents, inability to concentrate, headaches, neck, back and shoulder pains, indigestion, tiredness, cold sores, stomach pains, diarrhoea, palpitations. These are early warning signs which suggest that pressure is building up, and if you're experiencing more than a couple of them frequently, take time out to think about your life. If you don't, and you allow yourself to remain in a perpetually stressed state, physically and mentally, you are on the road to disaster.

Keep a diary of your thrush attacks: do they coincide with the onset of your stress reactions? Does each attack of thrush make you feel very depressed? After you've felt very stressed, do you have an attack of thrush? Talk to other thrush sufferers – believe me, nearly every woman you know will have suffered from thrush at some time in her life – and ask them if they feel the same way about thrush as you do. Then you can judge whether or not your stress could be getting out of hand.

Becoming assertive is a positive response to stress. Say what you mean, even if by doing so you hurt someone's feelings. It's you that's important. Saying you're fed up, you don't like something and you're not going to do something is far healthier than bottling up your true feelings, doing things you don't really want to do and so experiencing destructive stress responses. Having time to yourself helps, too – time when you can think, and relax, and try to understand why you feel the way you do.

Orthodox medicine has nothing to offer you if you're suffering from stress. Tranquillizers dull the senses, don't get to the root cause and are dangerously addictive. If you can't identify and remove the cause of the stress, you've got to learn to lower your arousal reactions, to increase your capacity to cope with it. A good way of doing that is to learn a relaxation technique. Relaxation helps the body to recuperate and the mind to cope. Being able to relax physically at will is the key to good stress management, and is a skill which has to be learned.

Hypnosis

Stage hypnotists have done much to cheapen what is a valuable form of relaxation. Hypnosis is not, as is popularly assumed, being put to sleep. Nor can a hypnotist make you do things you don't really want to do. A hypnotic trance is merely an altered state of consciousness which can best be likened to that pleasurable state of deep relaxation you feel when you wake up in the morning, realize it's Sunday and you don't have to get up, and sink back into your pillow in a blissful state of peace.

The art of self-hypnosis is best taught by a hypnotherapist, but it will only take a little practice for you to master the technique. It's not dangerous, and while you're in a light trance you can come out of it any time you want – if the phone or the doorbell rings, for example – and contrary to popular belief, everybody is capable of being hypnotized.

Hypnotherapists use varying techniques – but probably none of them will use spinning watches! You might be asked to concentrate on an image in your mind, or stare at a point in the ceiling. You might be asked to close your eyes or find they close involuntarily as relaxation washes over you. Then the hypnotherapist can talk you through the stages of hypnosis down into a trance.

The hypnotherapist can help you to relax initially by talking you through various muscles in your body, asking you to clench them and then relax them, until eventually you feel your tensions and stresses departing and your body unwinding. Your conscious mind will also be relaxed to such an extent that the hypnotherapist can communicate suggestions to your subconscious – suggestions that will enable you to relax and cope with your stress more easily in the future.

Each time you go through this routine, either with or without a hypnotherapist, relaxation should become easier and easier. Some hypnotherapists make tapes during their sessions so you can play them at home each day, and eventually you should be able to relax immediately you hear the hypnotherapist's voice. Soon you should be able to relax on your own, and develop the technique of self-hypnosis.

One form of self-hypnosis is to first relax yourself as much as you can by lying in the 'corpse' position on the floor of a warm room – that is, on your back with your legs and arms slightly apart, palms raised.

Working up from the feet, tense and then relax every part of your body, finishing with the head and face. When you are in a deeply relaxed state, start slowly breathing and counting rhythmically. Breathe in to the count of one, breathe out and say to yourself, go to sleep. Count like this until you reach ten, and by then you should be in a light trance.

Lie there and keep repeating to yourself, I am relaxed, I am happy, I am confident. Feel your stressful feelings disappearing. Visualize yourself lying on a warm sandy beach with the waves lapping at your feet and the sun shining down. Feel the warmth of the sun. Lie there for as long as you want just letting these good, positive feelings wash over you.

Then think about you, not as a stressed, worried person, but as a confident, relaxed person who is able to deal with crises calmly and who looks forward to each day with optimism. Picture yourself as that person: if one of the things you are stressed about is your relationship with your partner, for example, picture yourself happy and loving with your partner. Hold that image and feel good about it.

When you feel you want to come out of your trance, count yourself back. Say to yourself: when I finish counting I will be wide awake and full of life, but feeling utterly relaxed and happy. Then slowly count down from ten down to one. With a bit of practice, you should be able to develop your self-hypnosis skills to such an extent that you will be able to relax within seconds. A bonus is that you can also change your negative attitude to a more positive one.

It's possible to buy relaxation tapes to listen to which will do the work for you. Relaxation for Living is a charity which offers a holistic approach to stress management. Their specially trained teachers run classes all over the country; these are a mixture of theory, discussion and practical work. They also run correspondence courses for those who are not within reach of a class, publish fact sheets, and sell very good tapes on relaxation.

Practice makes perfect. If you spend half an hour a day practising self-hypnosis you should become so proficient that wherever you are – on a bus, a train or at the theatre – and you start feeling your stress responses are getting the better of you, you should be able to switch into it. Eventually, you should be able to handle the stresses that enter your life in a more appropriate way, and should find your health improving as a result.

Meditation

There are various forms of meditation, but they usually involve a series of techniques which calm your mind, change your awareness and help bring your thoughts under your own control, rather than letting your thoughts control you. Because meditation increases your awareness, you can recognize the early stirrings of stress and cope with them, and eventually you should find that meditation can infuse your everyday life with a tranquillity hitherto unknown.

Meditation has the opposite effect on your body to the fight or flight response – instead of speeding it up, it slows it right down. When you meditate, your heart rate and blood pressure decrease. Your breathing slows, your muscles relax and your metabolism slows. Your body goes into a state not unlike hibernation, and the benefits are almost incalculable: transcendental meditation is even starting to be recognized and recommended by many doctors as a valuable relaxation technique.

Meditation takes many forms and like hypnosis, works best if it is practised regularly. It is probably best to learn a meditation technique from an expert, although you can adapt one for yourself: a good book to help you is *The Complete Relaxation Book* by James Hewitt (Rider).

Set aside two periods of 20 minutes each day and find a quiet place where you won't be disturbed. Take the phone off the hook. Sit in a chair or cross-legged on the floor, but don't lie down as you might fall asleep: the object is to stay alert.

Once you're comfortable, start to relax. Close your eyes and take deep breaths, feeling the tension in your body dissolve. Then repeat to yourself a word or a phrase that you like – a mantra – each time you breathe in. The best known mantra is Om, but you can say anything. Instead of repeating the mantra you can, if you prefer, stare without blinking at an object – try a lighted candle – for about a minute and then close your eyes, concentrating on the image and keeping it in your mind for as long as you can.

After about 20 minutes, gently bring yourself back to your surroundings, open your eyes and stretch your body. You should feel relaxed and happy.

Yoga

Yoga is not just an ancient system of spiritual development. It is a popular and effective form of relaxation and self-help care, and can actually help prevent disease by maintaining bodily harmony.

Yoga concentrates on three aspects: breathing, meditation, and posture, and great emphasis is placed on proper breath control: practitioners of yoga believe that tension is often a result of incorrect, shallow breathing. Hatha Yoga, the most popular form of yoga taught in the West, consists of a series of postures which you hold for as long as you feel comfortable.

Yoga can become a way of life. The slow, controlled breathing yoga teaches together with the postures which keep the body flexible, tone up the internal organs and increase the circulation, and have a calming effect on body and mind. Yoga can also restore bodily harmony and build up the body's immune system so that it is able to fight off infection.

Complete beginners should seek out a local class to learn basic postures which can then be practised at home. Books can help, but it's best to learn initially from an experienced teacher.

> 'I felt really run down, particularly when I was premenstrual. I was getting first cystitis then thrush – it seemed as though it was happening every other month. Then someone persuaded me to go to a yoga class and I feel like a new person – calmer and more relaxed. I don't think it's coincidence that the thrush and cystitis seem to have gone.'

ANN, 41

Learning to relax can literally revolutionize our lives. It can have such a beneficial effect on our mental well-being that our physical health can improve, too. In the following chapter, we will see how we can achieve optimum health by strengthening our immune system – vital if we are to keep thrush at bay.

Chapter 7

STRENGTHENING YOUR BODY'S DEFENCES

AS WE HAVE SEEN, yeasts are normally present in all of us, and when the immune system is functioning properly, they pose no threat to health. But when the immune system is weakened, the yeasts start to thrive and grow, producing toxins that can cause health problems. It follows, then, that if we concentrate on strengthening our immune system we can keep thrush at bay.

The immune system is the body's defence mechanism. It's the immune system that helps the body recognize germs or any other invading matter, and eventually neutralize and expel them. When you have a sore throat, for example, the soreness isn't caused by the bacterium which is responsible for your throat infection, but by your body's defences fighting it.

If our bodies are threatened by potentially harmful invaders like viruses or harmful bacteria – antigens – the immune system swings into action by making antibodies, protein molecules which bind to specific targets to counteract them.

Our bodies are capable of producing a huge range of antibodies. Every bacterium that threatens us has its own appropriate antibody, and the body carries on producing them until there are enough antibodies to defeat the infection. If your immune system is strong and your body can produce antibodies quickly enough, they can kill the invader with the help of the white blood cells, and often the disease can be stopped without treatment. Immunization is based on this principle: dead bacteria is injected into the body, and this stimulates the production of antibodies which will be able to destroy invading bacteria of the same type.

A strong immune system enables you to remain in good health, as you then have the ability to fight off potential germs and viruses without drugs. If your immune system has been weakened in any way, your body hasn't got enough defences to fight off illness. There is a growing number of doctors who believe that the post-viral syndrome, Myalgic Encephalomyelitis (ME), could be triggered off by a weakened immune system.

We all know people who complain that, come the winter, they seem to get one cold after another: that's because they have a poor immune system. If a person develops AIDS, their immune system is so seriously impaired that they can't fight off illness at all, and victims usually suffer one infection after another before finally dying of a disease like pneumonia or cancer. An allergic person is one whose immune system is so hypersensitive that their body produces antibodies to substances that are not actually threatening, like pollen, or food, or dust, and it's the antibodies produced to deal with these 'threats' that cause the allergic reactions.

The yeast organism that causes thrush shouldn't normally be a problem to a healthy body, as once it tries to go beyond the areas in which it naturally lives, the immune system should attack and destroy it. But when the body's immune system is weak, it can't control the yeast and so it grows unchecked and starts to spread to other areas. Not only that, but if you're making life as comfortable as possible for the yeast by consuming a high-sugar diet and wearing snug-fitting nylon underwear, it's easy to see how thrush can keep on coming.

Way of Life

Often you may not even be aware that your immune system is weak. A lot depends on the sort of life you lead and where you lead it. Immune systems become impaired for a number of reasons, not the least being the pressures involved in 20th-century living. Pollutants, lead, nutritional deficiencies, junk food, food irradiation, food additives, antibiotics, tobacco, alcohol, and allergy-inducing substances including food, pesticides, and drugs: these all place great strains on our bodies and make our immune systems work even harder. No wonder some can't cope.

Stress can severely damage your immune system. Deficiencies of vitamins B_2, B_5 (pantothenic acid) and B_6 can lead to decreased antibody production, and the white blood cells which help dispose of invading bacteria become less active when B_{12} or folic acid levels are low.

So if you live on a busy main road where the air is highly polluted with lead-filled petrol fumes; if you have a stressful job and find it difficult to relax; if you smoke and drink a lot of alcohol and live on junk food, your immune system is almost certainly impaired.

It's also possible to inherit a weak immune system. If your mother didn't eat a nutritious diet when she was pregnant, or if she suffered from a lot of infections which weakened her own immune system, or if she drank a lot of alcohol and smoked heavily, this could have an effect on your own immune system.

How do you know your immune system is weak? One indication could be if you seem prone to minor infections like colds, sore throats or thrush. Your immune system can also be weakened by allergies, but it's possible that some sufferers of food allergies aren't even aware of it. An allergen is obvious if the allergic reactions are instant and severe – like rashes, or swellings, or wheezing or vomiting – but 'hidden' allergies, or food intolerance, which have started to be identified as the cause of a much wider and less specific range of symptoms (of which the over-growth of *candida* is but one), can be much harder to pinpoint. The only clue is often a general feeling of malaise and a susceptibility to infection.

'For three years I was getting regular attacks of thrush and they'd clear up after I used nystatin and then the thrush would return again with monotonous regularity. It was like being on a treadmill.

75

Eventually, in despair, I took a friend's advice and went to see a naturopath. She talked to me about my diet and general way of life and suggested I try an anti-*candida* diet for a while which included avoiding all yeast-based and fermented food – and no sugar! It was hard sticking to it but I persevered, and I've only had one thrush attack in eighteen months, and that was after I went on holiday and forgot about healthy eating!'

MELISSA, 34

There can be no doubt that our desire for fast, convenient foods which have been artificially coloured, preserved and flavoured to look and taste appealing has contributed to the ever-increasing number of people suffering from mild or severe food allergies. Many food manufacturers, wise to the fact that people are becoming concerned about eating what amounts to a chemical cocktail, have taken to labelling their products as being free from artificial colours and flavours. Then you read the labels carefully and discover that they contain other additives such as synthetic antibacterial and antifungal preservatives, high levels of sugar or salt, emulsifiers or stabilizers.

Food Additives

There are around 3,500 different food additives in use and each year more are introduced. It is now widely accepted that certain food dyes, particularly the yellows E102 (tartrazine), E104 (Quinoline yellow), E107 (Yellow 2G) and E110 (Sunset yellow) and the reds E122, E123, E127 and E128 can cause severe allergic reactions in sensitive people and provoke hyperactivity in children. The preservative E223 reduces the vitamin (B_1) content of the food to which it is added, and the preservatives E245-252 are suspected of being carcinogenic. It's not surprising, then, that a diet consisting largely of processed foods can significantly weaken your immune system.

Of course, not all convenience foods are loaded with chemicals, but sometimes it's hard to sort out what's what, as additives can be hidden and therefore are not listed on the packaging. What we believe to be healthy, unadulterated food can often turn out to be the opposite. Take fresh salmon. On the face of it, there can scarcely be a more healthy and natural food. But if that salmon was reared on an intensive fish farm it might have been fed food which includes a banned food dye which is known to cause eye damage in humans, to give it its distinctive pink colour. Yellow dye is sometimes included in the feed given to battery hens to make their egg yolks a brighter yellow. Cattle are often given growth hormones and antibiotics, and residues of these can still be present after the animal is killed. So without knowing about it, we could be consuming a diet dangerously high in toxins.

The Pill

When someone has a kidney or a heart transplant, the biggest fear doctors have is that their body will reject the new organ. After all, the body regards a transplanted organ in much the same way as it regards a germ or a virus – as a hostile invader, and so it musters all its defences to get rid of it.

To stop this happening, potent immuno-suppressant drugs are given for some time afterwards to suppress the body's natural immune system. These drugs are steroid hormones, which are produced in increased amounts naturally during pregnancy, and which also form the basis of the contraceptive pill. It follows, therefore, that taking the Pill for a long period of time can have a devastating effect on your immune system.

Surgery

Surgery severely depletes the body of nutrients, particularly vitamins C and E and iron, and after surgery it is important to build up your immune system not only by eating a highly nutritious diet, but also by taking supplements. Don't take supplements after surgery without guidance, however: see your doctor or a nutritionist.

Strengthening the Immune System

Many things strengthen our immune system. Probably the most important is good nutrition in the form of a diet rich in fresh vegetables and fruit, unrefined carbohydrates, vitamins and minerals. But also important are the air that we breathe, the water we drink and the type of food we eat.

Polluted air pushes up our need for nutrients and puts great strain on our immune systems. So does drinking water loaded with chemicals. Stress debilitates our systems, can seriously impair our immune system and pushes up our needs for nutrients. Alcohol in large quantities robs the body of precious vitamins including vitamin C, which is vital for maintaining the immune system. So does smoking.

If you are a stressful person, either learn to manage your stress in a positive way and make it work for you or learn a relaxation technique (see chapter 6). In an ideal world you should be able to boost your immune system merely by adopting a nutritious diet and relaxation, but we don't live in an ideal world. Most of us don't want to live a nun-like existence, cutting out everything from our lives that isn't utterly good for us, and anyway, it's not possible to live anywhere that is free from pollution. The fall-out from the Chernobyl disaster affected the most unspoilt, remotest and previously unpolluted areas of the world most of all. None of us can escape pollution. So boosting your immune system by taking regular supplements of minerals and vitamins has to be a good idea.

But first, take a look at the food you eat. It doesn't take much to switch to as natural a diet as possible. A diet high in refined carbohydrates which supplies a less than adequate supply of vitamins and minerals can impair the immune system and encourage thrush to recur. Merely replacing refined foods like sugar, white bread, pasta and rice with wholefoods – wholemeal bread, wholewheat pasta and brown rice – can do a lot to repair the damage.

Drink skimmed milk instead of whole milk: that way, you take in all the vitamins but not the fat. Eat fresh fruit and vegetables instead of tinned, and if possible, eat organically grown food – that is, eggs, vegetables, fruit, bread and meat produced without the aid of artificial fertilizers, pesticides or feed additives. Often pesticides and fungicides are absorbed into the produce itself and can't be washed out.

Organic produce can be expensive if you buy it in supermarkets. If you can't grow it yourself, try and buy direct from the grower: there are lots of small organic farms around which sell direct to the consumer at reasonable prices. Organic meat can be hard to find, although bigger supermarkets are starting to stock it and big cities often have a butcher who sells only free range meat.

Some of our tap water contains a high level of harmful nitrates, and most tap water has added fluoride to which some people can be allergic. Questions are starting to be asked about the long-term safety of fluoride. Many people prefer to drink bottled water, or to invest in a water filter to reduce the harmful chemicals like aluminium and to bring down the chlorine level in the water.

Alcoholic drinks are generally bad news if taken in excess, because apart from the obvious adverse effects too much alcohol can have on you (long term liver damage and stomach ulcers, to name but two) many drinks, especially lagers and wine, contain chemical additives. Red wine contains chemicals called 'congeners' which can be responsible for a range of allergic symptoms, so it's better avoided altogether. Don't forget that all wine is produced using a process of fermentation using yeast, so it may aggravate a recurrent thrush problem.

Even fresh, unadulterated food can cause allergies in sensitive people. Common allergens are coffee, milk, wheat products, alcohol, nuts, chocolate and fruit juice, and often people don't realize that these are causing them to feel unwell. As we've seen, hidden food allergies can be notoriously difficult to pinpoint, especially when the symptoms are vague and not specific.

If you suspect you are allergic to or intolerant of a particular food, it's easy to test for it. Just cut the food out of your diet for a month and then gradually introduce it back into your diet. If you start feeling unwell, or if you get an attack of thrush, or if you just don't feel as healthy as you should do, the chances are you're allergic to the food, or have an intolerance.

If you think you might be allergic to something but don't really know what, the only way you can really find out is to go on an elimination diet. The most commonly used elimination diet involves consuming only lamb, pears and Malvern water (apparently the least allergic foods there are) for the first five days, gradually introducing other foodstuffs to see what is causing the allergy and then establishing a balanced diet. It requires great motivation: Action Against Allergy (see the appendix for address) can help. Your doctor may recommend you to a clinical ecologist, who specializes in the diagnosis and treatment of food allergies. Be cautious about going to a clinical ecologist unless you have been recommended or referred. Some can charge very high fees for their services.

If you discover a particular food is giving you all sorts of unwelcome symptoms, it's obviously not a good idea to have it as your staple diet. You might be able to enjoy it occasionally, however: if you are eating a well-balanced, nutritious diet, you're healthy and your immune system is strong, you should be able to eat the odd 'danger' food. It's when you eat it the whole time that the rot sets in.

Supplements

Vitamin and mineral supplements are not substitutes for food. We cannot stop eating, take vitamins and hope to remain healthy. What taking supplements *can* do is to back up a nutritious diet and so help fight infection. How much you need to take depends on your way of life. One person's requirement for specific nutrients may be as much as ten times more or less than another's: a stressful person whose job involves regular contact with pollutants will need to take more supplements, for example, than a relaxed person who works on an organic farm. We also vary in the way we use and absorb nutrients, depending on the amount of anti-nutrients to which we are exposed.

Although taking a good multi-vitamin supplement won't hurt

you, it's advisable to seek advice from a trained nutritionist or reputable complementary medicine practitioner before taking high doses of vitamins, as very high doses can lead to unwelcome side-effects.

Among the nutrients which are essential to keep the immune system healthy are the antioxidant nutrients – vitamin C, beta-carotene, selenium, vitamin B_6, and vitamin E – whose job is to protect the body from disease. They are 'free radical' scavengers – that is, they can play a vital role in removing free radicals, which are created as by-products of oxidation and can cause tissue damage.

An antioxidant is a substance which can prevent or delay oxidation of a molecule, and vitamin E is a protector whose primary function is the protection of the health of the body cells; taken as a long-term supplement, it can protect against damage from ozone which is present in smog, particularly in hot weather. Oxidation caused by ozone in smog can damage the immune system. Dosage is usually between 200 and 400 IU (international units) a day.

Vitamin C is the other important nutrient which taken in high enough quantities (around 1000 – 3000mg a day) can increase the production of antibodies to strengthen the immune system, and it also protects against infection. In large doses it can stimulate the immune system, and it therefore plays an important part in healing tissue and can help clear up a thrush attack more quickly. Furthermore, taking large quantities of vitamin C every day can acidify your system and so provide a hostile environment for *candida*.

Vitamin C is a water-soluble vitamin, which means the body does not store it and so it needs to be taken on a daily basis. However, avoid taking high doses of vitamin C if you are taking the contraceptive pill, because it can counteract the effects of the pill as it alters the way our bodies absorb oestrogen. If you are under severe stress, it has been shown[1] that large daily doses of vitamin C can maintain high levels of adrenal cortical hormones in the blood, which can actually impair rather than boost the immune system.

Beta-carotene is converted to vitamin A by the body, and is best taken naturally – from dark green leafy vegetables, carrots and some yellow fruits. Don't take vitamin A supplements unless it's under supervision, as taken in too high a dose, they can build up to toxic levels.

'After I read about vitamin C protecting against colds I started taking regular 1000mg doses throughout the winter and not only did I go through the entire winter without a cold, I didn't have an attack of thrush, either – the longest I'd gone without one.'

SUE, 32

Vitamin B_6 is especially helpful for women when the balance of the hormones can be upset during the pre-menstrual period. It helps make antibodies to fight infection, and can counteract the adverse effects of the contraceptive pill. Take it in a vitamin B-complex tablet daily.

The Nature's Best company produce a supplement called Imuno-Strength which contains herbs such as Echinacea and Devil's Claw, vitamins and minerals, which support the body's defences naturally. They have also recently brought out a supplement, ImuGuard, which is based on active immunoglobulin concentrate: immunoglobulins are proteins with specific antibody activity against antigens. Another 'all-in' supplement which saves you the trouble of working out your own nutritional needs is Health+Plus Ltd's Detoc Formula II, an 'anti-pollution' food supplement which provides the nutrients which help neutralize the pollutants found in so much of our food nowadays. The Solgar company in New York produce an excellent multivitamin and mineral supplement called VM-75 which, taken daily, should help build up your immune system.

Having strengthened your immune system by sticking to a highly nutritious diet, trying to pinpoint allergens, avoiding pollution and learning to cope with stress, in the following chapter we shall now look at the role diet can play in actually causing thrush – and how it can help contain it.

Chapter 8

YOU ARE WHAT YOU EAT: THRUSH AND DIET

W E'VE SEEN IN CHAPTER 7 that if we live off a diet high in refined carbohydrates and low in nutrients, our bodies won't receive enough fuel in the form of vitamins and minerals to remain healthy: eventually our immune system will be impaired, and we will become less and less able to ward off illness.

We have also seen how various outside influences like stress, pollutants, drugs, and smoking can push up our demand for nutrients, making it even more crucial that we eat a nutritious diet.

And we know that a poor diet can not only predispose us to thrush by weakening our immunity, but certain foods – even highly nutritious, healthy ones – can actually aggravate thrush because they cause the yeast to thrive.

A diet high in yeast-promoting foods like beer, wine, cheese, and bread can, combined with a high sugar intake, encourage the thrush organism to grow even without any other precipitating factor.[1] If you have recurrent thrush which seems to be impervious to all else, it could be that you need to change your diet radically if you want to eliminate candida. *Candida Albicans: Could Yeast Be Your Problem?* by Leon Chaitow (see Further Reading, page 121) explains how yeast overgrowth can be controlled by depriving it of its nutrients, as well as strengthening the immune system using a strict dietary regime.

Whether or not you feel you need to completely rethink your eating habits, diet is of the greatest importance in not only helping to eradicate thrush, but also in controlling it and helping to ensure that it doesn't recur.

Of course it's unrealistic to expect that any active woman who might well have a full-time job as well as having to run a home has the time or inclination to prepare freshly-cooked food at every meal. There are times when even the most zealous followers of nutrition and diet buy a convenience food or TV dinner.

Besides, what is a convenience food? A loaf of bread? A bottle of tomato ketchup? A jar of pickles? Few of us have the time to bake our own bread or make our own pickles and sauces. The occasional ready bought meal or takeaway won't hurt us. It's when we consistently skip meals, snack on crisps and chocolate instead of eating properly balanced meals, fill ourselves up with fizzy cola drinks, and only ever eat TV dinners that we start running the risk of becoming undernourished.

A low-fibre diet high in salt, refined carbohydrates like sugars and white flour, processed foods, alcohol, and fats can lead to a build up of intestinal toxic bacteria. These can destroy the beneficial bacteria which keep the harmful bacteria and yeasts in check. Constant dieting, or crash starvation dieting, can slow down your metabolic rate and lead to less cell replacement and building. And that means an impaired immune system, which leaves you open to illness, and lack of energy.

A balanced diet should provide carbohydrates, proteins, vitamins and minerals. This means meat, fish, eggs, beans or lentils; milk and other dairy products; unrefined cereals, fruit, vegetables, butter, margarine and oils.

A sufficient intake of protein is vital to remain healthy. We need a regular intake of protein in the form of beans, pulses, grains, meat, fish or dairy products for the repair, replacement and growth of cells and tissues. Fats provide energy, and small quantities are needed to repair the body's wear and tear, and growth of tissues. Fats are either saturated or unsaturated: the former usually come from animals and increase cholesterol level in blood, and the latter from vegetable sources. Carbohydrates are foods which contain carbon, hydrogen and oxygen and are anything sweet or starchy – sugar, biscuits, bread, potatoes, root vegetables, cereals. They are eventually converted into sugars, and unrefined carbohydrates are a good source of energy.

How you cook and store food is important. You might pride yourself on your diet which you think is high in nutrients. But the way you treat your food might be responsible for its nutritional content all but fading away.

Vitamins leach away if you chop up vegetables and leave them sitting in water for hours; if you overcook vegetables (better to steam than boil. Better still, eat raw vegetables); if you don't put lids on saucepans; if you leave milk standing in the sun; if you store fruit and vegetables for long periods of time, even if it's in the fridge; if you peel most vegetables (notably potatoes); if you add bicarbonate of soda when you cook vegetables to keep them green; if you fry; if you cook vegetables in too much water.

Fibre is the material in certain foods that is not digested in the alimentary tract and is then excreted by our body. It is only comparatively recently that people have realized how essential fibre is to our good health, and that the lack of fibre which has become such a characteristic of western diet, has been responsible for a sharp increase in diseases of the gut. It is fibre that is responsible for the swift passage of toxic substances from your system.

Prior to this discovery, food manufacturers went to a great deal of trouble to remove fibre from staple foods like bread. This has meant that a generation has grown up with the taste for bland, smooth refined foods like white sugar, bread, rice and pasta, from which most of the goodness has been refined. Nutrients lost refining wholewheat flour include vitamin E, vitamin B_6, iron, potassium, and zinc to name but a few. Too many refined foods put a great strain on the gut, and toxic levels of waste can build up as there is little or no fibre to propel the waste on its way out of the body.

So refined and convenience foods often have much of their vitamin and mineral content depleted, as well as their fibre. They haven't got an awful lot going for them nutritionally. But worst of all as far as thrush sufferers are concerned, they very often contain high levels of sugar.

Sugar and its Relationship with Thrush

Refined sugar is a completely unnecessary food. It gives you energy, as do all carbohydrates, but it's an empty energy: because sugar provides none of the vitamins and minerals we need to keep healthy, after the quick 'hit' you get from consuming it, you're left hungrier and with less energy than before. We can also get that energy from other sources: a piece of wholemeal bread will give you the same amount of energy as a spoonful of sugar.

On average, we consume the same amount of sugar in two weeks as we used to in a year 250 years ago. Half the sugar we eat is taken in tea and coffee; most of the rest is hidden in products like biscuits, jams, sweets and cola (7 spoons per can) so that we are not even aware we are consuming it. A small tin of baked beans and a tin of tomato soup, for example, contains the equivalent of two spoonsful of sugar. Sugar also comes in many forms – sucrose, the refined sugar which is also found in honey, fructose, which is fruit sugar, and lactose, which is milk sugar.

Too much sugar can cause diabetes, which in itself is linked with thrush. As we have seen, the walls of the vagina are kept lubricated by secretions. These secretions contain glycogen, or sugar, and the friendly bacterial flora which lives in the vagina, *Lactobacillus acidophilus*, transforms this sugar into lactic acid. The lactobacilli are responsible for keeping the *candida* organism from getting out of control in the intestines and also for the acid environment of the vagina: a diet high in sugars not only compromises the immune system, it can also mean that the lactobacilli won't be able to keep up with such a high level of sugar. Not only that, but yeast thrives on sugar. So the yeast will start to grow, the lactobacilli will start to diminish and *candida* will gain a foothold. No wonder thrush keeps recurring!

Yet another reason for avoiding a low-fibre diet is because such a diet encourages a rapid release of sugars into the bloodstream. This could cause extra high levels of insulin to be released from the pancreas to cope with it. Insulin enables the body to use the sugar by increasing the rate at which the sugar is withdrawn from the blood and into the tissues: too much insulin could cause the blood sugar levels to drop too low – a condition known as hypoglycaemia, which can sometimes signify diabetes. Uncontrolled diabetes can precipitate thrush.

> 'I noticed that I often got an attack of thrush when I had premenstrual tension, which for me was usually characterized by an addiction to chocolate which manifested itself in incredible binges when I'd eat maybe half a dozen bars. It wasn't until I started taking nutritional advice and changed and supplemented my diet that the cravings stopped and so, more or less, did the thrush.'
>
> MARIE, 35

Hypoglycaemia, which is characterized by feelings of tiredness, confusion, faintness and hunger, can develop if you habitually eat low-fibre, starchy, sweet food, and drinking alcohol, tea or coffee at the same time makes it worse. Sometimes people with a severe candida overgrowth can have cravings for sugar or sweet foods. It can be a vicious circle: you get a craving, and eat something sweet; the sugar makes the yeast grow, and the more it grows the more it uses up the sugar you're providing – thus lowering the blood sugar. Eating sweet foods relieves it, but only temporarily. In the end it merely exacerbates the problem because it leads to more insulin being produced, and so on.

Starving the Yeast

Candida flourishes on a diet high in refined carbohydrates. All carbohydrates are broken down into simple sugars as they are digested, and eventually changed into glucose which is used for energy. Refined carbohydrates have all the fibre and most of the nutrients removed, so only the starch remains – to be converted quickly into sugar.

Unrefined carbohydrates in the form of wholegrain bread, cereals, rice and root vegetables are not only high in nutrients and fibre and so are helpful in re-establishing your beneficial intestinal flora, but the process of converting the starch into sugar is slower, which means your system isn't suddenly overloaded with huge amounts of sugar.

As thrush thrives when you have a high blood sugar level, follow a low-carbohydrate diet and eat plenty of fresh fruit and vegetables, protein in the form of meat, fish, eggs, beans or lentils, dairy products but not too much fat. Avoid cakes, sweet drinks, sugar: if you can make it past the first week without putting sugar in your tea and coffee, you'll be able to appreciate what tea and coffee really taste like – and wonder how you could have ever wanted to mask their delicious flavour with sugar.

If you suffer from persistent thrush, it might be worthwhile experimenting for a month cutting out fermented foods, foods containing yeasts, fungus and refined carbohydrates (white flour, white pasta, white rice, cooked peeled potatoes) and sugar. This should starve the yeast and stop it from multiplying, and if you build up your beneficial bacteria as well, your immune system will be better able to resist the yeast getting out of control again.

This means no bread which contains baker's yeast, although you can eat soda bread or wholemeal pitta bread instead. No cakes or biscuits; mushrooms; cheese (except ricotta or cottage cheese); soya sauce; fruit and vegetables which are bruised or mouldy; grapes; dried fruits (they are high in sugar and often contaminated with mould); alcohol; B-vitamin supplements containing yeast; yeast spreads; vinegar; pickles, chutney and ketchup; sugar, molasses, honey, malt, jam, ice cream, puddings, sweets and candy; fizzy drinks; baked beans including sugarless brands; tinned soups.

Garlic

In chapter 5 we saw how garlic, as a powerful natural antibiotic, can be used to give symptomatic relief from thrush attacks by inserting it into the vagina. But garlic's antibacterial and healing qualities are so important that if you eat some each day, it should help protect you against thrush. I couldn't do without the copious amounts of garlic I add to just about everything from salad dressing to stew, but some people don't share my enthusiasm – and it does make you smell pretty ghastly the following day. So hooray for odourless concentrated garlic supplements, which you can buy from health shops. Taken daily, they are a powerful protectant.

You will find much more detailed information and recipes in Richard Turner and Elizabeth Simonsen's *Candida Albicans Special Diet Cookbook* (see Further Reading section).

It might be worth having a good clean-out of your food cupboards. If yours are anything like mine, they contain bottles of dried herbs and spices which date back years. Throw them away! These often gather yeasts and moulds during storage. Use fresh seasonal herbs instead.

Yogurt

The normal intestinal flora is made up from groups of micro-organisms including *lactic bacteria*, or *lactobacilli*. These are very important, as their work in transforming sugar into lactic acid creates a favourable environment which arrests the development of toxic bacteria including *candida*, and protects the intestinal mucus against the invasion and activities of harmful micro-organisms. *Lactic bacteria* are also able to produce certain B complex vitamins.

One way of building up your *lactobacilli* to protect you from an invasion of *candida* in the gut or the vagina is to take *acidophilus* supplements or fermented milk like kefir or live yogurt. We've seen what a marvellously useful product yogurt can be, for not only can it be used to relieve the symptoms of thrush, it's also an invaluable way of building up your *lactobacilli* either by putting it straight into the vagina during an attack or just eating it every day, which will help stop thrush from recurring.

Live yogurt – which is quite different from the well-known branded stuff you can buy in supermarkets – can be hard to find. You can make your own quite easily and cheaply, thus ensuring that you have a constant supply.

It helps if you have a yogurt maker, but it's not essential. You'll need a pot of live yogurt to start off your culture, and two pints of milk. Bring the milk to the boil and then let it cool to 75°C (so you can just about bear to hold your finger in it). Stir in two tablespoons of the yogurt culture and either cover the container with a plate and leave it in a warm place overnight, or pour the yogurt into a thermos flask. It should be set within 24 hours: then you should put it into the fridge to inhibit further bacterial growth. It should be ready to eat 12 hours later. Save a pot of the yogurt and you can start the whole process off again, and never be without some. Having a constant supply of yogurt on hand is essential for a persistent thrush sufferer.

Chapter 9

ACUPUNCTURE AND BODILY HARMONY

T RADITIONAL CHINESE MEDICINE is based on a completely different way of thinking from western medicine. The Chinese believe that illness comes from within, and they maintain that our good health is determined by our ability to maintain a balanced internal environment. Western doctors believe the reverse and yet paradoxically, acupuncture is one form of alternative medicine that is rapidly gaining acceptance by our orthodox medical profession.

Acupuncture can treat thrush very effectively, and can play a major part in preventing it from recurring. It can restore the body's natural harmony and help keep infection at bay. It can help us remain in good health and can even relieve symptoms. It has been shown to be especially useful for pain relief, so it can help during a particularly bad thrush attack when you feel swollen and itchy. It is also a useful way of treating cystitis, thrush's close partner in crime, and can break the wearisome thrush/cystitis circle. And apart from all that, it can strengthen your immune system and improve your general health.

The Chinese believe that we all have a life force – or 'Ch'i' – which circulates through us along invisible channels or pathways called meridians. When this flow of energy is disrupted, we become susceptible to illness.

An important part of Chinese medicine is the acceptance of the principle of opposite influences – Yin and Yang, the qualities of energy that control our health and well-being. They are complementary in the same way as left and right, dark and light, heavy or light, and just as there can be no left without right, there can be no Yin without Yang. The parts are interlocking and cannot operate on their own, and when we are healthy, there should be an absolute balance of Yin and Yang in our bodies.

Our bodily organs are either Yin or Yang: Yang is associated with stimulation, heat, wind, dry, hardness, activity, light; Yin is associated with cold, stillness, softness, wet, sleep, darkness. Another important factor are the Five Elements, or Phases – Fire, Wood, Earth, Metal, and Water, which are linked with the seasonal changes. The primary characteristic of each phase is determined by what happens in the natural world during each season, and each of the Five Elements govern a pair of meridians, one Yin and one Yang.

Our vital life force depends on the harmonious interplay of these natural forces, and they are constantly fluctuating according to the changing seasons. If they become unbalanced – if there is too much Yin, for example – we might upset the balance of our body, our Ch'i starts to circulate unevenly or even becomes blocked, and our body can become sick.

Many things can disrupt the flow of the Ch'i: stress, poor nutrition, surgery, climatic factors like extreme cold or heat, or damp; overwork, imbalances in diet or lifestyle. Since a yeast overgrowth can occur when the natural balance of the body or its immune system has been upset by antibiotics, poor nutrition or stress, acupuncture can be a useful form of therapy to use, especially in conjunction with symptomatic treatment like herbal compresses or douches (see chapter 10) to relieve the most irritating symptoms.

The Chinese believe that when you are sick, you show either Yin or Yang symptoms. If the symptoms are 'cold' – if you are very pale, for example – it's a Yin complaint. If you are hot or feverish, it's Yang. The object of acupuncture, therefore, is to rectify the imbalance, correct the disruption and create a harmonious balance of Yin and Yang by stimulating or sedating specific points along the meridians.

Acupuncture is not normally used to cure the symptoms, although it can alleviate them. It aims to restore and maintain the balance in the body, mind and spirit. An important part of the treatment is you: for the treatment is based on the belief that we all have natural self-healing powers, and all acupuncture does is to stimulate these powers.

There are 12 main meridians along which our life force flows, and these correspond to different organs of the body – heart, spleen, lung, kidney, liver and pericardium (which has no western equivalent) which are yin, and small intestine, stomach, large intestine, bladder, gall bladder and triple burner (again, this has no western equivalent) which are Yang. They each have various numbers of acupuncture points associated with them.

The organs are paired together in Yin and Yang couples through their channels, and each pair is linked with one of the five elements. These bodily organs give each other mutual support.

Practitioners insert the needles in particular points along the meridians to stimulate or sedate these points, either to get the Ch'i flowing or to sedate it. The skill lies in being able to locate the exact point: a good acupuncturist will be able to locate them exactly. As the meridian is often some way from the affected organ, where the acupuncturist puts the needle might seem unrelated to the actual complaint.

'I was having acupuncture treatment for stress which I'd been suffering from very badly. One of the visits happened to coincide with an attack of thrush and I mentioned this. The acupuncturist told me that the two things were related but that he could also do something about the thrush. That was a year ago and I haven't had an attack since. It could be a coincidence, as I don't have a problem with stress anymore. Or it could be the acupuncture. Whatever, I'm happy.'

JOAN, 43

Diagnosis is important in acupuncture. If you go to an

acupuncturist because you have been suffering from recurrent thrush, you might be a little surprised when he or she questions you about your way of life and family history, asks to see your tongue and feels your pulse.

This tells the acupuncturist a lot about your general state of health, and a good acupuncturist can learn a lot about your flow of energy and discover any imbalances there might be just from pulse diagnosis. He might ask you about your sleep patterns, whether you prefer hot or cold temperatures, what sort of food and drink you like, what sort of work you do and the sort of life you lead. He will probably give you advice about your diet and lifestyle. Not until the acupuncturist has made a thorough diagnosis will he be able to decide where your energy imbalance is, and work out which points needs to be stimulated or sedated.

He carries out a thorough diagnosis because an important principle of acupuncture is to get to the root of the problem. Not until this has been identified can the treatment be decided upon, for it is from there that the disharmony emanates. Next, the balance of Yin and Yang must be restored, and then the Ch'i is strengthened. Practitioners insert the needles in particular points along the meridians to stimulate or sedate these points to get the Ch'i flowing or to sedate it.

The needles are very fine and they don't usually hurt when they are inserted, although you might be left with a bruise afterwards. They are inserted at varying depths, according to where the points are, and might then be moved around depending on the treatment. Then they're left in for anything up to twenty minutes. During this time you can feel wonderfully relaxed – many people go to sleep. Stimulation can also be done electrically, or with heat, which involves burning herbs or 'moxa' in a cup on the needle, or on a stick. How many treatments you need depends on your state of health.

'I would come away from each treatment feeling so relaxed and feeling so good I could hardly wait for my next visit. And because I felt like that I felt my confidence grow and when that happened,

I felt strong and healthy. It was almost as though I was becoming fitter with each treatment.'

GILL, 36

Traditionally, acupuncture was used not only as a cure but a preventive: traditional Chinese acupuncturists used to visit their patients regularly not to cure them but to keep them healthy – and they didn't get paid if their patients became ill! We in the west are only now beginning to realize the great benefits of preventive medicine, along with a healthy lifestyle.

Acupuncture is not an instant cure. Some people become very impatient because often they can't see results for a while, but it can take time for bodily harmony to be restored. Although often you can see early signs of recovery, sometimes you can feel worse before you feel better.

Acupuncture can work well in helping to defeat thrush, because not only can it help your body back to health, it can ensure it *stays* healthy. It can be a valuable aid to relieving the symptoms of stress, possibly because it can reduce the levels of adrenalin for which stress is responsible, and it can stimulate the body's natural painkillers. Together with an improved diet, many thrush suffers have reported an almost miraculous cure rate after being treated with acupuncture.

Everyone has the potential to respond to acupuncture, but because there is no universal treatment, how well it works probably depends more on the practitioner than anything else – although you play a pretty big part. So, as with all alternative therapies, make sure you see a reputable practitioner.

Shiatsu and Acupressure

Acupuncture should only be performed by a qualified acupuncturist – it is one of the few natural therapies which shouldn't be attempted by the lay person. But there is an alternative therapy which is based on similar principles to acupuncture and is, in effect, acupuncture without the needles: acupressure, which you can practise on yourself and which is a good alternative to acupuncture for children or those who have a phobia about needles.

It is similar to a Japanese therapy called shiatsu which has lately become popular in the west. The object in both is to stimulate or sedate the life force, or Ki as it is called in Japan, at various points along the meridians using finger pressure or massage. The main difference is that whereas shiatsu involves pressure with elbows, knees, and hands, acupressure only uses finger pressure. It can either be used as a sort of massage over certain areas to stimulate the flow of energy, or else using the fingertips to stimulate specific acupuncture points.

For massage, read stretching and pressure, not the knead and slap variety you find at health clubs. As with acupuncture, disease is regarded as the result of the life force being unbalanced, and the practitioner aims to help your own healing processes and self-development; working directly with the body and your energy enables him to discover the underlying causes of a condition. The shiatsu itself doesn't do the healing: it stimulates your mind and body to heal itself.

You've probably performed a sort of shiatsu on yourself before: how many times, for example, have you had a period pain and rubbed your stomach or back to try and get some relief, or massaged your aching muscles, or pressed your hands over your temples when you've got a headache – and felt better? A shiatsu practitioner would maintain that you felt better because you've stimulated your vital energy to heal yourself.

Shiatsu is also a valuable stress reliever and can be used to induce a state of relaxation. It's also good if you're convalescing after an illness, as it can help build up your immune system, and it can be used to ward off disease. It can help to prevent thrush because it keeps you healthy by restoring and maintaining your bodily harmonies, and stimulating the flow of body fluids and energy. You can learn basic techniques from a teacher and practise on yourself quite safely. After or even during a shiatsu or acupuncture session, it's not unusual to feel a bewildering array of feelings and emotions as your bodily energies are stimulated. You can feel incredible feelings of euphoria.

Many practitioners of traditional Chinese medicine use herbal medicine in conjunction with acupuncture. Herbal medicine, which dates back many thousands of years, is the basis for modern medicine. In the following chapter we'll be looking at various forms of herbal medicine and how it can help thrush – both symptomatically and as a preventative.

Chapter 10

THE HEALING POWER OF HERBS

Herbalism

HERBALISM IS AN ANCIENT SYSTEM of natural medicine which prevents and cures disease using the roots, stems, seeds and leaves of plants and herbs. Our remote ancestors instinctively sought out plants with healing properties, and healing herbal remedies have been handed down from generation to generation. Modern medicine owes a lot to herbalism and many drugs are derived from herbal remedies: heart drugs from digitalis, or foxglove; morphine from the opium poppy.

But herbal medicine today is more than just an array of potions made from natural ingredients, which are dispensed to give symptomatic relief in the same way as is orthodox medicine. It is based on a holistic approach to health. It can be used to relieve and treat the symptoms of thrush, but the medical herbalist will not just prescribe an ointment to stop the itching, or a medicine to clear up the discharge. Like other alternative practitioners, the herbalist regards disease as a sign that the body is trying to heal itself, and so merely suppressing the symptoms is not enough. The root cause must be discovered.

Therefore, a herbalist will build up a picture of your whole lifestyle and general health and take a full medical history before prescribing, and he will tailor his treatment to your individual needs. Like the acupuncturist, his aim is to assist natural healing and to restore the balance of your health.

If, for example, you have been suffering from recurrent thrush and cystitis, it could indicate a degeneration of the tissues of the urinary system, and that will need treating and strengthening before your health can improve. If you have been suffering from thrush as a result of a hormone imbalance, herbal medicine can be very effective in not only encouraging hormone production but in repairing damaged tissues.

Herbal medicine can be potent. You cannot make up your own remedies, although there are some symptomatic treatments – infusions, herbal compresses and douches – which you can make up. Some health shops sell herbs, although specialist herbal shops usually sell the best range, and they have the added bonus of being run by a herbalist, whose advice you can seek.

Even drinking herbal teas such as camomile, which can be bought from health shops, can soothe inflammation, and symptomatic relief from thrush can be had using herbal compresses and infusions. A compress can be made by wrapping herbs (fresh ones are best) in a piece of damp cotton and wearing them as a pad until it dries out. Try golden seal, sage, myrrh, comfrey, thuja or camomile. Calendula is an effective anti-fungal.

Herbal infusions can be made by pouring a pint of boiling water over an ounce of dried herbs or ground-up root (using a mortar and pestle) or 3 oz of fresh herbs. Leave it to steep in a china teapot for ten minutes or so and then drink a cupful up to 3 times a day.

Some women have found vaginal douches made from golden seal (a teaspoon to a pint of warm water) are effective, although douching tends to be more popular in the United States and Europe than in Britain. Douches should not be used often, as regular douching can actually upset the balance of the vagina and precipitate more attacks of thrush. They should also not be used before, during or just after a period, or during pregnancy. Great care should be taken (see page 115 for further information on douching). An alternative which many women prefer to douching is to soak a sponge with the solution and put it into the vagina.

We've already seen that garlic, which plays an important part in herbal medicine, is a versatile powerful natural antibiotic and antiseptic. A clove of peeled garlic put into the vagina for a night either wrapped in a piece of cotton so you can remove it easily, or with a piece of thread through it, can relieve the symptoms. You can also make an infusion of boiled, chopped and peeled garlic. When it's cool, you can either use it to make a compress and wear it as a pad, as above, or bathe your genital area with the solution, or dip a tampon in it and leave it in the vagina overnight. Garlic is a safe and healing herb.

If you're lucky enough to have a garden you can grow your own herbs, but take care if you gather herbs from the wild. Have a herbal book with you if you're in any doubt, because some poisonous plants look very like some herbs. It's probably safer and easier to buy from a herbalist. If you keep dried herbs, store them in a dark cupboard in airtight jars and write the date on which you bought or bottled them on the jar. Herbs can go mouldy after a while, and if you use mouldy herbs you could set off an attack of thrush.

Symptomatic relief can be obtained by bathing the vulva with a few drops of tea tree essential oil (see section on Aromatherapy on page 103) diluted in a little water, and cotton wool pads soaked in witch hazel will soothe an inflamed vagina.

Homoeopathy

This is a system of natural medicine based on the principle that like cures like – that is, the remedies prescribed induce in a healthy person symptoms which they cure in a sick person. It's rather like x-rays: a small dose can cure cancer in a sick person, but too much can actually cause cancer in a healthy person.

Homoeopathy has been around since the days of ancient Greece but was only rediscovered at the beginning of the last century by a German doctor, Samuel Hahnemann. He noticed that quinine, which was used to treat malaria, produced malaria-like symptoms when it was taken by a healthy person. He therefore decided that the symptoms of the malaria weren't the disease itself but the body's attempts to combat illness, and that we are capable of fighting off most illnesses ourselves. By suppressing the symptoms with drugs, we are denying our body the chance to cure itself.

Homoeopathy stimulates the body's defence system and allows it to overcome the disease naturally. The principles behind it are similar to those of vaccination: introduce a small quantity of the organism that causes disease into the body, and this stimulates it into producing its own defences against it. Dosage is crucial: dosages are more potent when given in lowest concentration or highest dilution. In other words, the smaller the dose, the better it works.

Homoeopaths also share the belief that disease is associated with lifestyle and is a result of often hidden, internal causes, and that if a cure is to be effected the whole person must be treated. If you visit a homoeopath he will build up a comprehensive picture of your way of life and general health, your emotional state and happiness, even find out what sort of childhood you had. The remedy he will then prescribe will match your own particular symptoms and characteristics: he won't just prescribe a remedy to cure thrush.

Often the condition can worsen before it gets better, but as soon as there is an improvement the remedy must be stopped. If you carry on taking the remedy longer than necessary, you can stir up the symptoms again.

True homoeopathic remedies are made up from many substances. Most chemists stock basic homoeopathic remedies: you can relieve the symptoms of thrush by making up a solution of 20 drops of tincture of calendula to half a pint of cool boiled water and bathing the affected area with it. A treatment for thrush is Helonias 6c, twice a day, but be sure to stop when the discharge clears. But to get the best results from homoeopathy, you should see a qualified homoeopath.

Homoeopathy is more closely aligned with orthodox medicine than any other alternative treatment, and many medical doctors practise it. There are even homoeopathic hospitals within the NHS in Britain. Your doctor should be able to refer you.

Aromatherapy

Aromatherapy is the therapeutic use of natural aromatic essences, or essential oils, obtained from the bark, flowers, plants, leaves, stems, and roots of aromatic or scented plants. Try taking a few spikes from a rosemary plant and rubbing them between your fingers: what you'll see is a tiny quantity of the plant's essential oils, and it will smell wonderful.

Aromatherapy can be practised through inhalation, massage or general application to the skin. It can be used in baths, or even taken internally, although that should only be done under supervision. It can be used for relaxation purposes, as a beauty treatment, for therapeutic reasons or to prevent illness from occurring.

We've seen how a weakened immune system can be responsible for persistent thrush attacks. Aromatherapy can help build up the immune system naturally. It can also alleviate stress and tension, fight infection, reduce inflammation and promote healing. The oils can be therapeutic even added to a bath.

Aromatic substances have a long history of healing. The ancient Egyptians used to use perfumed oils in medicine, which they obtained from adding crushed bark and distilled flowers to oils. Special gardens were planted along the banks of the Nile specifically to grow medicinal plants. These plants were gathered from all over the world, and the anti-bacterial qualities of their essential oils were recognized, as they used them to embalm their dead. During the Great Plague in Britain in the 17th century, aromatic substances like pine were burned in the streets and it was common for people to carry aromatic pomanders to protect them from infection.

Early this century, a French doctor rediscovered the healing powers of oils and they were used to treat injuries in the first world war. His work was taken up by an Austrian biochemist, Marguerite Maury, whom most aromatherapists regard as the modern pioneer of aromatherapy. She developed a treatment which mainly consists of massage.

Aromatherapy is increasingly being recognized as having a

valid place alongside orthodox medicine. In France, where the medical efficacy of aromatherapy has long been recognized, an aromatherapist must also be a qualified doctor. Unfortunately, elsewhere anybody can set up as a practising aromatherapist so it's wise to visit an aromatherapist on recommendation. But it's a treatment that lends itself to self-help as well.

It is often thought of as a beauty treatment, but many therapists are interested in aromatherapy as part of a wide spectrum of holistic medicine, and aim to help patients maintain a balance of mental, physical and spiritual health.

Aromatherapists take into account the mind, body and spirit of the person as well as lifestyle, eating patterns, environment and relationships. Some aromatherapists embrace the Chinese idea of the complementary opposites Yin and Yang, when all bodily energies are in a state of balanced, perfect harmony. So although it's a treatment you can carry out yourself, like other forms of natural medicine, you'll derive the best benefits if you see a qualified practitioner.

If you have any doubts about the therapeutic value of essential oils, think about how good you feel when you smell scented flowers. Why do we fill our houses up with bowls of potpourri? It's because the essential oils they emit have a therapeutic effect on us. They alleviate anxiety and depression. They make us feel happy.

It's most important to use only high quality natural essential oils – not synthetic chemical essences, which will not have the same properties. Indeed, how the essential oils are extracted from the plants is important and will influence the therapeutic properties of the oils – even what time of the day or night the plant is gathered. Synthetic essences are ineffective for medicinal purposes and may even be harmful if used other than as a pleasant-smelling bath additive.

Aromatherapy can be used for local treatment – that is, by putting the oils, suitably diluted, directly onto the afflicted part. Certain essential oils help reduce inflammation and work well in treating soreness and bruises, and they have been shown to affect the body's hormone-producing glands. But aromatherapy is best used, like all holistic medicine, as a preventive.

In Britain and the United States the essential oils are usually administered via massage, although you can add them to baths or inhale them. The neat oil must first be diluted with a vegetable oil such as cold-pressed olive oil or almond, in a concentration of 1-3% of essential oil to base, or the oil can cause irritation. It's best not to take essential oils internally except under the supervision of an aromatherapist.

Some essential oils are sold ready diluted: check before you buy. Price is usually an indicator: diluted oils will be cheaper than concentrated oils. A whole body massage will probably need about 25ml vegetable oil with between 8 – 12 drops essential oil. 20 drops of essential oil equals 1ml.

The action of massage, whether it's done by a professional, a friend or your partner, can be wonderfully healing, physically and mentally. It can activate the nerve endings and stimulate the circulation, and it eases the entry of the oils into the body tissues.

The oils should be massaged firmly into the skin without squeezing and you should relax as much as possible, as the oils will not enter a tense body. Absorption takes between 10 minutes and an hour and a half, depending on the essential oils.

Oils can also be added to a warm bath: ten drops of diluted oil per bath. This is a good way to absorb the oils as not only can you absorb them through your body, you can also inhale their vapour in the steam from the bath, if you keep the doors and windows shut. Don't have the bath too hot, or the sweat from your body will prevent the oils being absorbed. You can make your own steam inhalation by adding five drops of oil to half a bowl of boiling water: put a towel over your head and inhale the vapour. That really makes you feel good.

Just as certain organs derive particular benefits from vitamins and minerals, so they do from essential oils. Lavender, myrrh and tea tree oil (which is a relatively new oil obtained by distilling the leaves of an Australian tree), all have anti-fungal properties. You can use them separately or a blend of all three, either in a bath or in a massage. Tea tree is quite powerful, and so could irritate the delicate membranes, so use it in slightly lower proportions than the others. Calendula is another good anti-fungal oil.

The oils can also be made up as a douche (see chapter 11 for information about douching). Six drops of tea tree mixed with a litre of warm water has proved to be beneficial for some women, as have rose, lavender and bergamot. Tea tree, as well as being anti-fungal, is renowned for its germicidal properties and is good for treating herpes as well as thrush. This should alleviate the itching, but don't douche for longer than a week because you could upset the natural balance of the vagina. If you don't like the idea of douching, use the solution to make a compress (see page 101) and wear it as a pad until it is dry. Some aromatherapists treat thrush with pessaries made from essential oils such as tea tree, which work well and are a lot more efficient, safer and less messy than douching.

Regular baths containing tea tree, juniper or lavender essential oils can help guard against recurrent thrush as these stimulate the immune system. In a massage use 7 drops tea tree, 7 drops lavender, 7 drops bergamot and 4 drops sandalwood in 50ml base oil.

Aromatherapy is completely safe, providing you follow a few basic rules. Don't take the oils internally unless prescribed by a qualified aromatherapist, as some can be toxic. Never use oils without first diluting them, as you could cause irritation. Don't use them for longer than three weeks as they might build up in your system and become toxic. Certain oils including sage, rosemary and myrrh should be avoided by pregnant women, and tea tree shouldn't be used if you have a sensitive skin or suffer from allergies, as it may have a skin sensitizing effect on some people. Don't use too much: the oils are highly concentrated (unless you buy them ready diluted) and you only need a tiny amount. Too strong a concentration can make your thrush worse and set off even worse itching and inflammation.

Genuine essential oils are quite expensive. Treatment by an aromatherapist is likely to be expensive, too, as sessions can be lengthy. Often reflexology foot massage is used by aromatherapy practitioners as part of the treatment. This is a holistic therapy which, like many other alternative remedies, is based on the belief that we have a life force, or energy, which flows through our bodies via channels. The body is divided into zones of energy and each channel relates to a zone and the organs in that zone. Congestion or tension in any part of the foot mirrors congestion or tension in a related part of the body, so by applying pressure to the feet you can relax and heal the whole body and restore its natural equilibrium.

Bach Flower Remedies

These are a system of 38 remedies derived from plants and devised in the 1930s by a medical practitioner turned homoeopath called Edward Bach. Bach came to the conclusion that the root cause of physical ailments was an emotional or mental problem. He believed that a negative frame of mind, coupled with an emotional problem, upsets the harmonious balance of our system, resulting in illness; not until you cure the emotional problem can you cure the illness. He worked out 38 negative mental and emotional states to which we are all prone, and the remedies, said Dr Bach, cover every state of mind known to humans.

The remedies work particularly well in conjunction with other forms of medicine, particularly homoeopathic, or even with orthodox medicine. These are not symptomatic remedies, as the object is to discover why your negative state of mind has occurred before it can be treated, and what remedy will work for you depends on your emotional make-up. The remedies can be bought from health shops or directly from the Bach Centre. They are completely safe to take internally, and are just one more option for you to try. For choice is what treatment is all about.

Chapter 11

KEEPING THRUSH AT BAY – FOR GOOD

I F YOU'RE PLAGUED by recurrent thrush, it can make you feel so fed up and wretched that it's often hard to think about anything else other than obtaining the quickest and most effective form of symptomatic treatment – which is almost certainly anti-fungal drugs. There's no doubt that they are effective. And because they usually bring swift relief, it can be easy to forget that the thrush can recur – until the next attack.

For as we've seen in the previous chapters, anti-fungals don't prevent thrush from recurring. They might stop the symptoms, but they don't solve the basic problem of why thrush occurs in the first place. That involves looking at your way of life, your general health and your diet. Restoring your body's natural equilibrium and strengthening your immune system is the best way of controlling thrush and ensuring it doesn't recur. But to give thrush as little chance as possible we'll take a last look at its predisposing factors, so that you don't give it even the tiniest chance to thrive. It might mean adopting a slightly different way of life – but isn't it worth it?

We have seen that there are certain times when we are most at risk from the invading yeast:

- during pregnancy
- after taking antibiotics

- if we eat a high-carbohydrate diet
- during the premenstrual period
- if our immune system is weakened for whatever reason.

Some women can see a definite pattern in their thrush attacks: it's a help to keep a diary to see if there is a specific trigger to your attacks. Then, if you know you are at risk – for example, if you are prone to a thrush attack at the latter end of your menstrual cycle – you can take precautions against thrush in the form of supplementation with live *Lactobacillus acidophilus*.

Contraception

IUDs increase your susceptibility to vaginal infection because of the string that hangs down from the uterus, which can become contaminated. The diaphragm also slightly increases your risk of thrush, because although it is usually flexible, a badly-fitting diaphragm can inflame the vaginal wall. And of course, if you leave a diaphragm in for too long, you can set up a nasty infection which can trigger an attack of thrush. Some forms of contraceptive pill, because of the hormonal changes associated with them, can precipitate thrush, although there is no evidence that this is the case with the low dosage pill.

Please don't throw away your usual form of contraception in a panic. But if you have recurring thrush, it might be worth looking at your method of contraception and perhaps switching to another method for six months, as an experiment. Changing your brand of contraceptive pill might help, or having your diaphragm checked to see if it is the right size. And remember to be extra vigilant about hygiene if you do have a diaphragm.

Sex

Your partner can be affected by your thrush. He can develop an inflammation of the penis called balanitis, or can have a hypersensitive reaction to the yeast. A condom does give him some protection, but it's best to avoid sex during a thrush attack.

Furthermore, you increase the risk of infection even more as the thrush might have been precipitated by an infection in the first place. Most women find the idea of sex during a thrush attack a turn off anyway. Thrush makes you feel unclean and anything but sexy.

It helps to have an understanding partner during attacks: it's hard enough coping with the threat thrush poses to our sexuality and self-confidence without being hassled by an insensitive partner. It's not a very good idea to switch to oral sex as a substitute, either, as there is a slight risk of your partner contracting thrush in his mouth.

Thrush can seriously affect your sex life, physically and psychologically. Imagine the scenario. You have sex while you have thrush. It is very painful, and the friction possibly makes the thrush worse. You are going to feel reluctant to repeat the experience, and next time your partner suggests sex, remembering how it felt the last time, you are unenthusiastic. If you do have sex, you are tense, expecting it to hurt. Eventually you could develop a phobia about sex which could even manifest itself as vaginismus, when the muscles of the vagina tense up and form a sort of 'no entry' sign to such an extent that the man is unable to insert his penis.

Unlubricated sex can cause abrasions in the vagina which can lead to thrush. If you have difficulty with lubrication, use a lubricating jelly like KY, not Vaseline.

Sometimes an attack of thrush can follow a sexual encounter with a new partner, particularly if you have led a relatively sex-free existence for some time before. This leads a lot of women to believe that they caught the thrush from their new man, whereas it's probably just a reaction to their new partner's sperm. If you've had a long time without sex and then suddenly start having vigorous and frequent sex with a new partner, this can be such a shock to the system that it can trigger a thrush attack.

Hygiene

Hygiene can help prevent thrush, particularly if you take a

hygienic regime on board as a way of life, not just during a thrush attack. Passing water and washing your genitals after sex can protect against thrush and cystitis. Wiping lavatory paper from front to back, and not the other way round, can stop *candida* from transferring from the anus to the vagina. Washing after each bowel movement is also a good idea, because of the high risk of transferring bacteria from the bowel to the vagina and urinary tract. Avoid bidets – they can help cross-infection. Make sure your partner keeps his genitals clean.

Clothing

We've seen that thrush loves the warm, dark, damp environment that is created by wearing tight jeans, close-fitting nylon knickers, tights, and leotards. Even sleeping in an over-heated bed complete with tightly tucked-in bedclothes can exacerbate thrush. It's no good not wearing such clothes during a thrush attack and then starting to wear them again the minute the thrush has gone. You're merely laying the foundations for thrush to recur.

If you're prone to thrush, the safest thing to do is throw away all your tight-fitting trousers, knickers, tights and leotards, and replace your bed clothes with a duvet. You might not like the idea of never wearing jeans again, but isn't that better than thrush?

'I just couldn't stop my thrush recurring even though I faithfully followed the regime my doctor told me about and even stopped wearing tights and jeans. Then I realized that an attack quite often followed the dancing class I went to once a week when I'd spend three hours or so in a tight sweaty leotard. I switched to wearing a baggy tee shirt and, cross fingers, I seem to be okay ever since.'

LORRAINE, 28

Damp swimming costumes also provide a wonderful breeding ground for the yeast organism. If you're the sort of person who likes drying off in the sun after a swim – don't. It's a bore, but the only way to keep thrush at bay is to change out of your wet swimming costume immediately you emerge from the water.

Which brings us to the subject of holidays. Many people have had their holidays ruined by a thrush attack because they've blithely flown off to foreign climes without giving thrush a second thought.

Sometimes just a change of climate can precipitate a thrush attack, particularly if you're going somewhere hot and sticky. If you're predisposed towards thrush, prepare for your holiday by taking live acidophilus supplements a month before you depart. This builds up your reservoir of friendly intestinal flora and is a good idea on two counts: not only does it ensure that you can repel any potential yeast invasion, it also guards you against the tummy upsets that are often so much a part of exotic foreign travel.

As we've seen, yeast loves heat and that's what holidays are all about. Try going knickerless as much as you can on holiday (not recommended on the beach, unless it's of the naturist variety!); loose bikini pants are better than a tight one-piece swimming costume. Take an emergency treatment kit with you consisting of cotton wool and witch hazel, to soothe inflammation, and Aci-jel (see page 53) to acidify the vagina. Don't travel in trousers, particularly if it's a long, hot journey.

Washing Your Underwear

Candida spores from vaginal discharge are deposited on your underwear during an attack of thrush, and once your underwear is contaminated it can be very hard to get rid of. The spores can be a source of reinfection, and ordinary domestic washing won't eradicate them. The only way you can sterilize your underwear effectively is by boiling it at temperatures over 80° C, soaking it in bleach for 24 hours, or ironing it with a very hot iron – none of which are very practical ideas, particularly if you like underwear made from delicate fabrics.

There is another rather more convenient way of sterilizing your underwear – in a microwave. Experiments have shown[1] that damp *candida*-contaminated underwear can be effectively sterilized by microwaving it on a high setting for five minutes, and this is an excellent idea, because not only does it kill the spores, it also protects delicate materials. It's important that the underwear is damp, however – it doesn't work on dry underwear. If you do that throughout the duration of an infection, it may reduce the risk of the thrush recurring.

Soaps, Deodorants and Bubble Baths

The cosmetic industry has made a fortune out of preying on women's fears about body odour. To be accused of smelling unpleasant is, to many women, one of the worst things that could happen to them; so terrified are we of body odour that we're lured into spending millions on deodorants, talc, soaps, perfumes, bubble baths, and body sprays in order to mask our perfectly natural bodily smell.

It was these fears that caused the manufacturers of vaginal deodorants to enjoy a short-lived boom in sales some twenty years ago after they were introduced. Fortunately, vaginal deodorants have now been recognized as not only unnecessary and, because of the implication that natural vaginal odour is in some way unpleasant, rather offensive. And as we've seen, vaginal deodorants can actually provoke thrush attacks because they can dry out and irritate the vagina, kill off the natural bacteria and even set off an allergic reaction. Vaginal 'wipes' or cleansing tissues can also have an adverse effect. Far better to use cotton wool and warm water if you need to freshen up.

Bubble baths and highly scented soaps can irritate the vagina and kill off the friendly bacteria, making the vagina vulnerable to abrasions. Never use soap to clean your genital area, unless it's pure and non-scented like Simple Soap. Flannels and sponges harbour germs unless they're boiled daily, so use a piece of cotton wool instead.

During a thrush attack, the best and most soothing way of cleaning yourself is with a piece of cotton wool soaked in pharmaceutical olive oil. Don't dry yourself with a towel, especially if you share it with a partner – use a hair dryer or tissues. And if you're an inveterate thrush sufferer who enjoys nothing more than a long soak in a boiling bath, it's a luxury you're going to have to forego, probably for good. Having hot baths exacerbates thrush as the organism loves the warmth. Stick to warm baths or showers.

Some biological washing powders and fabric conditioners can cause irritation in susceptible people, and if you're a thrush sufferer it might be worth experimenting with different washing powders. Even coloured lavatory paper has been known to irritate sensitive vulvas, so stick to white, preferably unbleached.

Keeping clean shouldn't mean masking our bodily smells with scent. A normal healthy clean vagina has a very distinctive smell, and it's not unpleasant. Many men find it a turn on – far more so than a vagina which is covered in chemically perfumed talc. Once you've got the confidence to accept that, you'll not only save a fortune in deodorants and bath additives – you'll discourage thrush, as well.

Before a Period

It's common for thrush to appear just before or during a period, because the pH of the vagina rises (i.e. it becomes less acidic) due to the alkalinity of the blood, providing an environment in which the yeast likes to grow. If you are prone to thrush attacks around the time of menstruation, a few days before your period is due each month you can help prevent a thrush attack by inserting Aci-jel (see page 53). Taking high doses of vitamin C (between 500 and 1000mg) can help acidify your system, and adding vinegar to your bathwater can help, as can bathing the vagina in a vinegar solution (one tablespoon of vinegar to a pint of warm water).

Regular douching in a solution of dilute (3 per cent) hydrogen peroxide (one teaspoonful to 8 fluid ounces of pure (filtered or bottled) water) has been found to be an effective preventive in cases of very severe chronic thrush. Make sure you get the right concentration of peroxide: a stronger concentration can be dangerous.

Douching is not popular in the UK and therefore it might be difficult to get hold of a douche bag, although it is perfectly acceptable in many other countries. It can be a useful occasional form of treatment, although prolonged douching can disturb the vaginal flora and actually end up aggravating thrush.

Take care if you use a douche. Don't have the bag higher than two feet, and it's better not to raise it at all. Just lie in an empty bath and gently squeeze the fluid into your vagina. Too much pressure could force fluid into the uterus. Never douche when you're pregnant, or just before, during or just after a period. Perhaps a safer way is to insert a tampon soaked in a peroxide or vinegar solution or yogurt.

Yogurt can also be put directly into the vagina: a teaspoonful a time every night for seven nights in the premenstrual period. I'm sure we all know by now that it must be *live* plain yogurt, and any containing fruit, nuts or anything else just will not do! Only live yogurt contains lactobacilli – they will build up your vaginal flora which will keep *candida* down. Taking live *acidophilus* supplements if you think you are at risk, or even crushing them and putting them into your vagina (don't do that if you're pregnant) can help. Eating live yogurt every day will also help stop thrush recurring.

Wearing tampons during menstruation can aggravate a thrush problem. Tampons left in for long periods or forgotten can cause the vagina to dry out or become ulcerated or set up an infection, so it's important to change them frequently. Better still, switch to pads when the flow is heavy or during the night when you won't be worried about them showing under your clothes.

Knowing Your Body

My doctor's toes curl when I mention the subject, but regular cervical and vaginal self-examination is a good way of keeping healthy, as eventually you will come to recognize the early signs of infection and can obtain treatment before it takes hold.

How many of you have ever actually studied your genital area? How many of you know what your vagina looks like? Have you ever held up a mirror and studied your vulval area, so you know what colour it is when it is healthy? If not, how can you recognize any sign of infection or inflammation? How do you know whether or not the secretions from your cervix are normal or a sign that something's wrong?

The answer is you can't, unless you look. Just as regular self-examination of your breasts can help you to detect any lumps, so examining your vagina and cervix can help you see early signs of any infection.

It's easier than it sounds – providing you're relaxed about it. The only tool of the trade you'll need is a speculum. This is a small instrument made from either metal or plastic which holds the walls of the vagina open, enabling you to see inside. A speculum can be hard to obtain, although some good chemists might sell expensive metal ones.

Many doctors are horrified at the idea of self-examination and regard it as an encroachment on their territory: after all, the more their patients know about their bodies, the less control doctors have over them. Doctors attached to family planning clinics tend to be more sympathetic and will probably not only let you have one, but also show you how to use it. Women's groups often run self-help groups aimed at teaching women self-examination, and this is a good way to learn: many sell speculums as well for home examination. The Women's Health and Reproductive Rights Information Centre (see page 123 for address) can supply plastic speculums by mail order together with detailed instructions on self-examination at a very reasonable price.

As well as a speculum you will need a good light – an anglepoise lamp is best, but a strong torch will do; a mirror; and something with which to clean the speculum afterwards, such as antiseptic soap. Some women find it easier to insert a speculum if it is lubricated with KY jelly: experiment and see how you feel most comfortable.

Obviously, it is better if a doctor or nurse shows you how to use a speculum, as they can tell you exactly what to look for. Some doctors believe in self-examination, while others do not. Only you know what sort of reaction you're likely to get if you ask your doctor for help! Most of us, however, probably aren't lucky enough to have progressively-minded doctors but with a little patience and trial and error, you should be able to do it yourself.

First, have a good look at the speculum and practise opening and closing it. You will see what looks like a long beak – these are the blades of the speculum, and you are going to insert them into your vagina while they are still closed. When you can open and close the speculum easily, get yourself comfortable on a bed or floor with your legs bent and apart. It's easier to see what's going on if you're half sitting, propped up with cushions behind you, and it's probably easier if you get your partner or a friend to help you by holding the light in the right position.

Hold the mirror up and have a look at your outer genitals, or vulva. Check that there's no inflammation, rashes, abrasions or sores. Lubricate the speculum if you want – many women find it more comfortable. It's also easier to insert if it's warm.

Holding the speculum in the closed position with the handles upward, gently insert it into your vagina. It's easier if you're relaxed and not resisting, but even so, many women find it hard to do for the first time, particularly as it can seem rather large if you've never seen one before. When the speculum is in place and feels comfortable, and you feel confident, open the blades and lock them open.

Adjust the light and look into the mirror. You should be able to see the vaginal walls and the cervix. The cervix should look pink and shiny with what looks like a dimple in the middle. This is the os and is the opening to the womb, and it is only big enough to admit sperm in or menstrual blood out. If you examine yourself at various times during your cycle you will be able to see the changes that take place – the cervix, for example, changes in colour and position depending on where you are in your menstrual cycle, and the mucus changes in consistency and colour. After a while you should be able to tell what is normal for you as far as your cervix and vagina are concerned.

When you have finished, close the speculum carefully to avoid causing any abrasions to the vagina, and gently remove it. If you are suffering from thrush, sterilize it by boiling it (if it's metal) or cleaning it in antiseptic (if it's plastic). Don't examine yourself if you are pregnant: in fact, a good rule is not to insert anything other than a penis into your vagina during pregnancy.

Keeping Healthy

We've seen how a diet high in refined simple carbohydrates can trigger off thrush, not only because a high sugar intake can feed the yeast but also because it can undermine our immune system. Improving your diet in the ways we've seen – that is, by eating more unrefined carbohydrates such as wholemeal bread, pasta and brown rice; cutting out sugar altogether, eating fresh fruit and vegetables and pulses, and avoiding processed and junk food – will help keep you healthy.

Cut down on the foods that tend to precipitate an attack of thrush – yeast-based products like Marmite, mushrooms, cheese, bread (eat soda or pitta bread instead) and alcohol. Manage your stress successfully with relaxation techniques and get a good night's sleep. Building up your immune system and keeping yourself healthy is the best way to ward off further thrush attacks.

Adopting a healthy way of life is probably the best way to stop thrush from recurring. It's not going to be easy, for thrush can be obstinately difficult to shift. But it's simply not enough to cure the symptoms and hope for the best. Conventional medicine can't stop thrush from returning – only you can do that. And the resources you have at your disposal, your own powers of healing, are helped by achieving a state of optimum health.

FURTHER READING

Acidophilus and Lactic Bacteria: Essential Companions for Human Beings, Dr E. Brochu (leaflet published by Quest Vitamins (UK) Ltd)

Acupuncture Therapy, Mary Austin (Turnstone Press, 1974)

The Alternative Health Guide, Brian Inglis and Ruth West (Michael Joseph, 1984)

Alternative Medicine, Dr Andrew Stanway (Penguin, 1986)

Alternatives to Drugs, Arabella Melville and Colin Johnson (Fontana, 1987)

Alternatives to Healing, ed. Simon Mills (Macmillan, 1988)

Antibiotics: The Comprehensive Guide, Dr Ian Morton and Dr John Halliday (Bloomsbury, 1990)

Aromatherapy A-Z, Patricia Davis (C. W. Daniel, 1988)

Aromatherapy for Women, Maggie Tisserand (Thorsons, 1990)

Candida Albicans Special Diet Cookbook, Richard Turner and Elizabeth Simonsen (Thorsons, 1989)

Candida Albicans - Could Yeast be Your Problem? Leon Chaitow (Thorsons, 1991)

The Complete Guide to Food Allergy and Intolerance, Dr Jonathan Brostoff and Linda Gamlin (Bloomsbury Press, 1990)

The Complete Relaxation Book, James Hewitt (Rider, 1989)

Conquering Cystitis, Dr Patrick Kingsley (Ebury, 1987)

Cystitis: The New Approach, Dr Caroline Shreeve (Thorsons, 1986)

Diet and Nutrition, ed. Dr Elizabeth Evans (Octopus, 1984)

E For Additives, Maurice Hanssen (Thorsons, 1987)

Everyday Homeopathy, Dr David Gemmell (Beaconsfield Publishers, 1987)

Everywoman, Derek Llewellyn Jones (Faber, 1982)

Everywoman's Medical Handbook, Miriam Stoppard (Dorling Kindersley, 1988)

From Woman to Woman, Lucienne Lanson (Penguin, 1990)

A Guide to Homeopathy, Sarah Richardson (Hamlyn, 1988)

How to Improve Your Digestion and Absorption, Christopher Scarfe (ION Press, 1989)

THRUSH

Hypnotherapy Explained, David Lesser (Curative Hypnotherapy, 1988)

Massage Cures, Nigel Dawes and Fiona Harrold (Thorsons, 1990)

Medicine: The Self Help Guide, ed. Dr Susanna Graham-Jones and Professor Michael Orme (Viking)

Meditation, James Hewitt (Hodder, 1984)

Mitton's Practical Herbal, F. and V. Mitton (Foulsham, 1982)

The Natural Family Doctor, ed. Dr Andrew Stanway (Century Hutchinson, 1987)

The New Our Bodies Ourselves, eds. Angela Phillips and Jill Rakusen (Penguin, 1989)

The Side Effects Book, Dr Trevor Smith (Insight, 1989)

Stress Relief, Sharon Faelten and Diane Diamond (Ebury, 1989)

Understanding Allergies, Mary Steel (Consumers' Association and Hodder & Stoughton, 1986)

Understanding Cystitis, Angela Kilmartin (Century Arrow, 1985)

Victims of Thrush and Cystitis, Angela Kilmartin (Century Arrow, 1986)

Viruses, Allergies and the Immune System, Jan De Vries (Mainstream Publishing, 1988)

Vitamin Vitality, Patrick Holford (Collins, 1985)

Woman, Claire Rayner (Hamlyn, 1986)

What Acidophilus Does, Don Rowell (Felmore Health Publications, 1990)

USEFUL ADDRESSES

UK

Action Against Allergy
23-24 George Street
Richmond
Surrey TW9 1JY

Health Education Authority
Hamilton House
Mabledon Place
London WC1H 9TX

Women's Health and Reproductive Rights Information Centre
52-54 Featherstone Street
London EC1Y 8RT

Women's Nutritional Advisory Service
PO Box 268
Hove
East Sussex BN3 1RW

Institute for Complementary Medicine
21 Portland Place
London W1N 3AF

Acidophilus and other supplements (mail order):
Nature's Best Health Products
PO Box 1
Tunbridge Wells

Kent
TN2 3EQ

Lifeplan Products Ltd
Elizabethan Way
Lutterworth
Leicestershire LE17 4ND

USA

Candida Research and Information Foundation
31111 Palomares Road
Castro Valley
CA 94552

American Academy of Environmental Medicine
2005 Franklin Street, #490
Denver
CO 80205 *or:*
PO Box 16106
Denver
CO 80216

Women's Health Advisory Service
PO Box 31000
Phoenix
AZ 85046

Vitamin Suppliers:
Natren Ltd
12142 Huston Street
North Hollywood
CA 91607

Australia

Allergy Association
PO Box 298
Ringwood
Victoria 3134

Women's Health Advisory Service
PO Box 1096
Bankstown 2200

Women's Health Care Association
92 Thomas Street
West Perth
WA 6005

REFERENCES

Chapter 1
1   Berg AO, Heidrich FE, Fihn SD. 'Establishing the cause of symptoms of women in a family practice' JAMA, 1984.
2   Rodin P, Kolator B. 'Carriage of yeasts on the penis' BMJ, 1976.

Chapter 2
1   Ramakrishnan S, Radstone D. 'Carcinoma of the ovary' BJSM, 1990.

Chapter 3
1   Rosenberg, MJ. Letter to BJSM (1989).
2   Singha HSK, Devendra SV. 'Local Therapy for bacterial vaginosis – an evaluation of metronidazole sponges' BJSM, 1989.

Chapter 7
1   Richardson J. *Stress, adrenals and vitamin C* (Old Dominion University, Norfolk, VA, USA).

Chapter 8
1   Truss, CO, *The Missing Diagnosis,* quoted in *Candida Albicans* by Leon Chaitow (Thorsons).

Chapter 11
1   Edward G Friedrich Jr MD LLD and Lou Ellen Phillips PhD. 'Microwave sterilization of Candida on underwear fabric – a preliminary report' JRM, 1988.

INDEX

abscesses 36–7
Action Against Allergy 80
acupressure 95–7
acupuncture 91–5
adrenalin 65–6
AIDS 74
air
 lack of 29, 112
 pollution 78
alcohol 75, 78, 79
allergies 74, 75–6, 79–80
animal testing 59
antibiotics 11, 19–21, 26, 33–4, 38, 51, 53–4, 109
antibodies 73–4
anti-fungal drugs 20–1, 23, 51–4, 109
aromatherapy 103–7
assertiveness 67

Bach, Edward 107
Bach flower remedies 107
bacteria 11, 14, 20, 26
 lactic 9–10, 21
 rectal 14
 vaginal 9–10, 14, 19, 20, 21, 26 see also thrush
balanitis 13, 110

Bartholin's cysts 36–7
bathing 12, 28, 105, 106, 114–15
 in essential oils 105, 106
 in vinegar solution 45, 53, 60
bergamot oil 106
beta-carotene 81, 82
bubble bath 28, 114

calendula oil 105
Candida albicans 9, 14–15, 17
carbohydrates 29, 78, 84–5, 87–8, 110
cervical cancer 36, 41–2
cervical erosion 34–5
Ch'i 91–4
children 12
Chinese medicine, traditional 91–5, 104
chlamydia 37–8
Chlamydia trachomatis 37
clothing 12, 29, 112–14
complementary medicine 55–9, 91–107
compresses 106
contraception 21–2, 77, 81, 82, 110

corticosteroids 24
couchgrass 26
crabs see pubic lice
cystitis 12, 14, 26–7, 42–3

damp living conditions 27–8
deodorant, vaginal 28, 114
diabetes 24, 86–7
diaphragm 22, 110
diet 11, 29–30, 36, 58, 75–7, 78–82, 83–9, 119
 elimination 80
 see also food
dieting 84
doctors 13–14, 45–54, 55–6, 117
douching 60, 100, 106, 115–16
drugs 55–6, 59, 77
 see also antibiotics; anti-fungal drugs

Escherichia coli 26
essential oils 101, 103–7

fabric conditioners 115
fats 84

INDEX

fibre 85, 86
fight or flight response 65–8
flannels 28, 114
food
    additives 76–7, 79
    convenience 84, 85
    cooking and storing 85
    labelling 76
    organic 79
    refined 78, 84, 85
    see also diet
fruit 78

Gardnerella vaginalis 39
garlic 34, 38, 45, 60, 88–9, 100–1
genital disorders 31–43, 46
gonorrhoea 41
guilt 47

Hahnemann, Samuel 101
herbal teas 100
herbalism 97, 99–101
herpes 35–6, 106
holidays 112–13
homoeopathy 57, 101–2, 107
hormone replacement therapy 10, 23–4
hormones 18–19, 21, 22–3, 27, 40, 77
hygiene 14, 26–7, 111–12
hypnosis 68–70
hypoglycaemia 87

immune system 9, 17
    strengthening 25, 73–82, 103, 119
    weakening 11, 14, 20, 21, 25, 27, 58, 63, 73–5, 110
immuno-globulins 82
immuno-suppressant drugs 77
inter-uterine device (IUD) 22, 110
itching 13, 59–60, 106

juniper oil 106

know your body 116–18

Lactobacillus acidophilus 9, 21, 34, 38, 45, 59, 86, 110
lactose 11
lavatory, going to the 14, 27, 112
lavatory paper 115
lavender oil 105
lice 37
lifestyle 59, 74–6, 109, 119

massage 96, 103, 105
Maury, Marguerite 103
meat 79
medical examinations 46–7
    see also self-examination
medicine
    herbal 97, 99–101
    holistic (complementary) 55–9, 91–107
    orthodox 55–8, 67–8
    traditional Chinese 91–5, 104
meditation 70–1
men 13, 25, 38
menopause 10, 23–4
menstruation 11, 18–19, 23, 110, 115–16
meridians 91–4
metronidazole 33, 39
milk 78
minerals 78
    supplements 80–2
monilia 9
myalgic encephalomyelitis (ME) 74
myrrh oil 105

non-specific genital infections 39–40
non-specific urethritis (NSU) 37–8

oestrogen 18, 19, 23, 40, 81
olive oil 28, 60–1, 114
organic produce 79
orthodox medicine 55–8, 67–8
ozone damage 81

pelvic infection 22, 38–9
Pelvic Inflammatory Disease (PID) 38–9
penicillin 20
pessaries 52–3
pesticides 79
pill, contraceptive 21, 77, 81, 82, 110
pollution 75, 78, 82
pregnancy 11, 22–3, 34–5, 106, 109, 118
protein 84
pubic lice 37

reflexology 106–7
Relaxation for Living 70
relaxation techniques 66, 68–72, 78
rose oil 106
rosemary oil 106

sage oil 106
sandalwood oil 106
selenium 81
self-examination 116–18
sex 12, 13, 18, 24, 25, 31, 33, 40, 110–11
sexuality 47
sexually transmitted diseases 12, 25, 31, 33, 36–8, 41
    clinics 49–50
shiatsu 95–7
smear tests 41–2
smoking 75, 78
soap 28, 114–15
speculum 117–18
stress 27, 36, 58, 75, 78
    handling 63–72, 78, 119

signs of 67
sugar 29–30, 86–8
surgery 77
swimming 12

taboos 10
talcum powder 28–9, 114
tampons 29, 40, 116
tea tree oil 101, 105
thrush
  causes 11, 12, 17–30,
    109–16
  emergency treatment
    kit 113
  infection rate 10, 12
  oral 12, 23, 24, 111
  symptoms 13–15, 31–2
  treatment 15
    drugs 11, 12, 19–21,
      45–54, 55–6
    self-help 59–61,
      68–72, 88–9
    see also diet;
      relaxation

techniques
  what is it 9–11
towels 28, 114
toxic shock syndrome 40
trichomonas (TV) 14,
  32–4, 39
Trichomonas vaginalis 33

vagina
  acidity 9–10, 11, 18–19,
    21, 23, 115
  discharges 18–19, 21,
    23, 32, 34, 39, 46
  healthy 17–18
  infections of 14, 19, 21,
    23, 24, 26, 31–43,
    53–4
  odour 28, 114
  sugar in 19, 23, 86–8
vaginitis 40
  anaerobic 10, 39
  non-specific 39
vaginosis, bacterial 39
vegetables 78

vinegar solution 45, 53,
  60, 115
vitamins 75, 77, 78, 85
  A 82
  B₆ 81, 82
  C 81, 115
  E 81
  supplements 80–2

wart, vaginal 36
washing clothes 113–14,
  115
water pollution 78, 79
witch hazel 60, 101
Women's Health and
  Reproductive Rights
  Information Centre
  117
yeasts, growth of 9–11,
  83, 86–8
Yin and Yang 92–4, 104
yoga 71–2
yoghurt 21, 26, 34, 38,
  45, 59, 116